Tooth surface loss

Tooth surface loss

Edited by

Richard Ibbetson*
BDS (U.Lond.) MSc (U.Lond.) FDS RCS (Eng.)

Andrew Eder**
BDS Hons (U.Lond.) MSc (U.Lond.) LDS RCS (Eng.) MFGDP (U.K.) MRD RCS (Eng.)
RCPS (Glas.)

*Professor of Primary Dental Care and Director of the Edinburgh
Postgraduate Dental Institute, University of Edinburgh
and
Honorary Consultant in Restorative Dentistry, Lothian Primary Care NHS Trust,
4th Floor, Lauriston Building, Lauriston Place, Edinburgh, EH3 9YW

**Visiting Professor and Director of Continuing Professional Development,
Eastman Institute for Oral Health Sciences,
University College London, 123 Gray's Inn Road, London WC1X 8WD
and
Honorary Consultant in Restorative Dentistry, Eastman Dental Hospital,
University College London Hospitals Trust
and
Specialist in Restorative Dentistry and Prosthodontics,
57a Wimpole Street, London W1M 8YP

2002

Published by the British Dental Association
64 Wimpole Street, London, W1M 8AL

ISBN 0 904588 66 1

Printed and bound by Dennis Barber Limited,
Lowestoft, Suffolk

Foreword

Although significant progress has been made in our understanding of dental caries and periodontal diseases, as well as the promotion of prevention as an active form of treatment, it is clear that the problems of tooth surface loss will be a major challenge to the dental profession in this new millennium.

With this in mind, the London Chapter of the Alpha Omega International Dental Fraternity organised a comprehensive continuing education course of lectures for dental practitioners on the topic of tooth surface loss under the chairmanship of Andrew Eder. The contributors were invited to prepare papers based on their original presentations for submission to the *British Dental Journal*, whilst additional articles were also requested and these were all published during 1999. As the management of patients who present with worn teeth can be so varied, this problematic area has previously only been superficially addressed in many texts. However, this multi-authored book has been able to bring together the contributions of many experienced clinicians, academics and teachers.

In summary, the text covers the problematic and multi-factorial aetiology of tooth surface loss and looks at detailed methods of assessment and treatment. The comprehensive section on treatment planning illustrates the problems of decision-making, using clinical cases to exemplify the points made and to emphasise the importance of maintenance in order to avoid or mitigate future failure.

I congratulate the editors and contributors for compiling this user-friendly and comprehensive work that will be invaluable to all students and clinical practitioners as an educational and reference text.

Sir Ian Gainsford
BDS (U.Lond.) MGDS FDS RCS (Eng.) FDS RCS (Edin.) FICD FACD
London, March 2000

Contents

Tooth surface loss: Editors' introduction

R. Ibbetson and A. Eder

Tooth surface loss is an important area of clinical dentistry. We are publishing a new series on tooth surface loss and on this page, the editors introduce the whole series.

Tooth surface loss can arise as a result of erosion, abrasion or attrition. These processes are rarely seen in isolation and often cause patients to seek help for problems of pain, altered function and compromised appearance. Individuals of all ages can present with the condition: in this series attention will not only be given to the older patient but also to younger individuals affected by pathological tooth surface loss which is well in advance of their chronological age.

Emphasis is given to presenting practical clinical techniques which should help dentists to identify the aetiological factors responsible for tooth surface loss and assist in planning and delivering appropriate patient care. The authors include not only restorative dentists but other specialists: this reflects the fact that the management of some patients will require inter-disciplinary care.

Management of individuals suffering from tooth surface loss remains difficult but developments in materials and techniques have made the delivery of restorative care easier. The central difficulties that will be addressed in the series are:
- The difficulties of diagnosis and prevention
- The difficulties of controlling tooth surface loss
- The difficulties of restoration.

Difficulties of diagnosis

The three types of tooth surface loss each have their own characteristic appearance. However, the wear of an individual's teeth is rarely from a single cause although one is likely to predominate. The articles in this series define the characteristics of each and allude to the significant difficulties that the clinician frequently encounters in determining the dominant aetiology. There is emphasis on the need for thorough histories supported by diet sheets and sometimes assistance from medical colleagues in determining some of the intrinsic causes of tooth surface loss.

Difficulties in controlling the tooth surface loss

Identification of the causative factors is imperative. This can prove difficult or even occasionally disappointingly impossible. In the latter instances the likelihood of controlling the destruction of the teeth is low. However, many of the changes that we may be asking our patients to make represent significant changes in habits or lifestyle. The difficulty in achieving this should not be underestimated: patients often will require considerable support, encouragement and advice. The series repeatedly emphasises the fundamental importance of prevention and the available measures that can be used.

There also remains the difficulty of detecting slowly progressive tooth wear. Study casts, indices and photographs are all helpful. However, as the teeth generally continue to erupt as they wear, small amounts of further loss of hard tissue remain very difficult to detect. This makes monitoring the effectiveness of any preventive measures equally difficult.

Difficulties of restoration

In previous decades patients suffering from marked tooth surface loss would frequently have been provided with multiple crowns and bridges to restore appearance and comfort. Such treatment is complex and generally highly invasive. Consequently there has therefore always been a tendency to defer its provision if at all possible, with the consequence that tooth wear was usually well advanced before definitive restorative treatment was commenced. Patients were probably also deterred from undergoing long complicated and expensive courses of treatment until it became absolutely essential.

Developments in dentistry mean that this approach is no longer the only one available. While traditional crowns and fixed and removable prostheses still have a significant part to play, many conservative strategies can now be used to provide restoration and protection for damaged teeth. The continued eruption of teeth as they wear creates a major restorative difficulty. If restorations are needed, space must be created to permit an aesthetic and occlusally stable result. A number of articles in the series will describe the ways in which the problem of lack of space may be minimised or overcome. These apply the results from more recent research and developments in clinical practice that have simplified many of the restorative procedures for both patient and dentist.

The series will discuss the following subject areas:
- The causes of tooth surface loss
- The prevention and control of wear
- The restoration of worn teeth using both fixed and removable prostheses
- Maintenance and monitoring
- Dealing with failures.

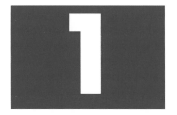

Tooth surface loss: an overview

M. Kelleher[1] and K. Bishop[2]

The management of tooth surface loss (TSL) demands a full understanding of its aetiology and presentation. This paper provides the introduction to the series and an overview of pathological, non-carious loss of tooth tissue. Emphasis is placed on the aetiological factors which are currently thought to be major causes of this problem. This directs the paper toward those agents that produce erosive tooth surface loss. This is appropriate given the increasing incidence and severity of this type of tooth wear.

The article attempts only relatively brief descriptions of the presentation and aetiology of attritional and abrasive tooth surface loss. This does not imply that they are less important but rather reflects the increased concern over the need for prevention, early detection and control of acid erosion. Later articles in the series will return to the presentation and management of the other types of TSL. The preventive management of bruxism is described in the third and sixth paper.

Non carious loss of tooth tissue is a normal physiological process and occurs throughout life.[1] If the rate of loss is likely to prejudice the survival of the teeth, or is a source of concern to the patient, then it may be considered 'pathological'.[2] The dental management of patients with such loss of tooth tissue has provided difficulties for the dental profession for many years and it is generally agreed that the problem is increasing. This can only partly be explained by the fact that the population is retaining more natural teeth into old age.[2,3] It is not only the middle-aged and elderly who exhibit pathological loss of tooth tissue, but also younger age groups (fig. 1).[4] Robb reported that the prevalence of pathological loss of tooth tissue in patients less than 26 years of age was greater than in many older age groups.[5] The *Child Dental Health Survey* (1994)[6] confirmed this when 32% of 14-year-olds had evidence of erosion affecting the palatal surfaces of their permanent incisors. This cannot be explained as an age-related phenomenon. It may, however, be the result of changing lifestyles and social pressures which have led to the increased prominence of particular aetiological factors.

Aetiology

Traditionally, the terms 'erosion', 'abrasion' and 'attrition' have been used to describe the non-carious, pathological loss of tooth tissue (Table 1). These terms reflect the specific

aetiological factors which are associated with the loss of tooth tissue. Eccles suggested that the term 'tooth surface loss' should be used when a single aetiological factor was often difficult to identify.[7] Smith and Knight, however, considered that 'TSL' belittled the severity of the problem and, therefore, advocated the use of the term 'tooth-wear' to embrace all three aetiological conditions.[2] Broad terms to describe the processes involved are helpful since a single aetiology is less common.[8,9] For clarity, 'TSL' will be used throughout this paper to describe the pathological, non-carious loss of tooth tissue although 'tooth-wear' and 'TSL' are often interchangeable. The terms, 'erosion', 'abrasion' and 'attrition' are still useful where there is a clear indication of a specific aetiology or where aetiological factors are being discussed.

Erosion

It would appear that erosion is a major cause of TSL. Smith and Knight, for example, could exclude it as a cause of TSL in only 11% of patients examined.[10] Traditionally, factors which may cause erosion have been described as originating from the following sources:[11]

- Dietary
- Regurgitation
- Environmental.

Table 1 Definitions of attrition, erosion, and abrasion

Attrition	The loss by wear of tooth substance or a restoration caused by mastication or contact between occluding or approximal surfaces
Erosion	The progressive loss of hard dental tissues by chemical process not involving bacterial action
Abrasion	The loss by wear of tooth substance or a restoration caused by factors other than tooth contact

Table 2 pH of commonly consumed drinks

Manufacturer	Brand	pH
Pepsi-Cola	Diet	2.95
Coca Cola	Regular	3.15
	Caffeine free – diet	3.30
	Tab clear – diet	3.20
Lucozade	Sport Orange	3.78
Tango	Diet Orange	2.80
Orange Juice		3.50

Pathological, non-carious loss of tooth tissue is an increasing problem to the dental profession, with young individuals especially at risk. This paper provides an overview of the problem with an emphasis on the possible causes, particularly those factors which may account for the increased incidence. The clinical appearance produced by the various aetiological factors is discussed and recommendations made on the objectives of the immediate and long-term management of the problem.

[1]*Consultant in Restorative Dentistry, King's Dental Institute, London;* [2]*Consultant in Restorative Dentistry, Maxillofacial Unit, Morriston Hospital, Swansea SA6 6NL*

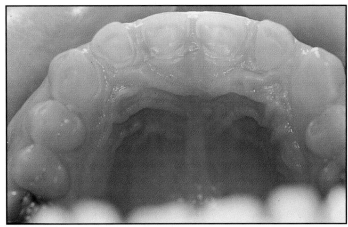

Fig. 1 Palatal view of maxillary teeth of a 16-year-old female who had drunk a litre of 'diet' carbonated drinks a day for the past two years. There is marked tooth surface loss affecting the anterior teeth, particularly the central incisors where the pulps are visible

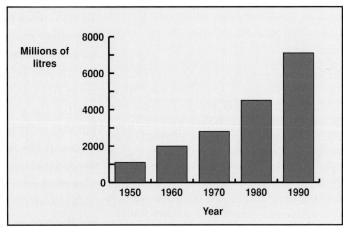

Fig. 2 Total soft drink sales in the UK 1950–1990
(Source: British Soft Drinks Association, 1994)

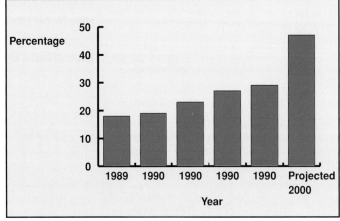

Fig. 3 Market share of 'diet' carbonated drinks in the UK
(Source: British Soft Drinks Association, 1994)

Dietary erosion
Dietary erosion may result from food or drinks containing a variety of acids, especially citric acid which may chelate as well as dissolve calcium ions.[12] Citric and phosphoric acid are common constituents of soft drinks and fruit juices (Table 2).[13] These beverages are now widely available, with a doubling of sales in the UK, since 1970 and a 7-fold increase since 1950 (Fig. 2).[9] Adolescents and children account for 65% of sales with 42% of fruit drinks consumed by children between the ages of 2 and 9 years old.[9,14] This consumption of soft drinks by this age group has been identified as the probable cause for the erosion recorded in the *Child Dental Health Survey* (1994).[6]

Slimness and 'healthy eating' are now perceived to be important in western society. This has helped the newer 'diet' drinks to achieve a greater share of the sales market (fig. 3). These low calorie drinks are also acidic (Table 2) with, except for the sugar, similar constituents to the traditional beverages. The potential for erosive damage by these 'diet' beverages may be less well appreciated. The acidic nature of soft drinks, therefore, makes them a significant aetiological factor in TSL, particularly in younger patients. Eccles confirmed the importance of these beverages when he reported that they were implicated as aetiological factors in 40% of patients with TSL.[15]

A 'healthy' diet may also contain substantial acidic foods[16–18] and cause further loss of tooth tissue. Furthermore, the abrasive nature of many of the components of these diets may accelerate TSL. (Certain dietary components, such as curries, also have the potential to cause TSL indirectly, by causing gastric reflux.[19])

Regurgitation erosion
Regurgitation results in gastric acid entering the mouth. The regurgitation may be involuntary or self-induced as in bulimia nervosa.[5,20]

Involuntary regurgitation: Involuntary regurgitation is a common complication of gastrointestinal problems such as hiatus hernia (fig. 4). The effect of the regurgitated acid on the teeth is well documented.[21,22] Furthermore, medication used to treat such problems may also be a cause of TSL.[22]

Gastritis and acid regurgitation are common complications of chronic alcoholism, although patients may not be aware of the problem.[23,24] Often the patient is secretive about the habit and confirmation is usually difficult. There is also a group of patients, for example the young adult, who have frequent alcoholic 'binges'. Such binges are often associated with episodes of vomiting. These patients tend to be less secretive about their alcohol consumption. Soft drinks which are frequently used as 'mixers' with alcoholic drinks may also contribute to TSL.

One of the major roles of saliva is to dilute and buffer any acid which enters the mouth and lubricate the occluding surfaces during mastication. If salivary flow is reduced, the potential for erosive and attritional damage increases.[25] As medical science advances and life expectancy increases, the use of drugs within the population is more widespread.[26] Many of these drugs cause a dry mouth and, as such, the associated problems are likely to become more prevalent.[27] The problem may be compounded if patients consume acidic drinks in an attempt to alleviate the symptoms and stimulate salivary flow.

Voluntary regurgitation:Voluntary regurgitation may be practised by patients with an eating disorder. Such disorders are a feature of a body-conscious society and often begin in early adolescence, frequently running a chronic course with substantial complications.[28] The prevalence of eating disorders in the general population would appear to be increasing with figures reported for anorexia nervosa of between 0.1–0.2% and 1–2% for bulimia nervosa. However, eating disorder patients may actively avoid detection or be reluctant to disclose details of their problem and as such the true prevalence may be underestimated.[28,29]

The effect of acid regurgitation in eating disorder patients has been well documented.[30–34] The most common sign is perimolysis — erosive lesions localised to the palatal aspects of the maxillary teeth (fig. 5). These lesions are thought to be the result of the tongue directing gastric contents forward during voluntary and prepared vomiting with the lateral spread of the tongue protecting the lower teeth.[16,32]

The pattern of TSL in eating disorder patients may also be affected by other aetiological factors such as:[16]
• Erosive 'diet' beverages and 'healthy' foods as patients strive to control their weight
• Xerostomia, caused by vomit-induced dehydration or drugs such as diuretics, appetite suppressants and anti-depressants
• Long-term complications such as gastric ulcers and hiatus hernia.[28]

Environmental erosion
Environmental erosion occurs when patients are exposed to acids in their work-place or during leisure activities.[35,36] Health and safety laws have probably reduced the risk of environmental erosion although it should not be ignored as a possible aetiological factor.

Environmental erosion predominantly affects the labial surfaces of the maxillary and mandibular incisors.

Attrition
Attritional TSL primarily affects the occlusal and incisal surfaces of teeth although slight loss may occur at the approximal contact areas (fig. 6). This type of TSL can be particularly significant in patients with a vegetarian or a modern 'healthy' diet.[37] Attritional TSL may also be a consequence of parafunctional activity.[38,39]

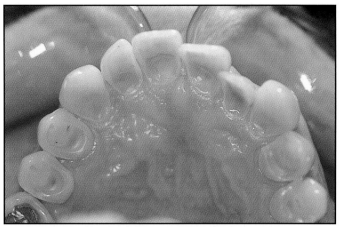
Fig. 4 Palatal view of maxillary teeth of a 35-year-old male with a history of hiatus hernia. There is general 'erosive' tooth surface loss, with the teeth having a rounded appearance with 'cupping' on the palatal cusps of the premolars. The damage is limited to the palatal aspects of the teeth

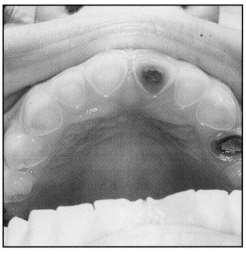
Fig. 5 Mirror view of the palatal aspects of the maxillary teeth of a 22-year-old female bulimic. Note the extensive 'erosive' tooth surface loss with the teeth having a rounded appearance and the surface characteristics lost. The 1| and 4| have been root-filled following pulpal necrosis

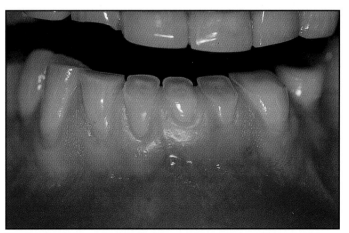
Fig. 6 Labial view of mandibular anterior teeth in a 40-year-old male bruxist. The teeth have flattened incisal edges as the enamel and dentine wear at the same rate. The teeth 'match' the palatal surfaces of the maxillary teeth in excursive movements

tooth surface loss

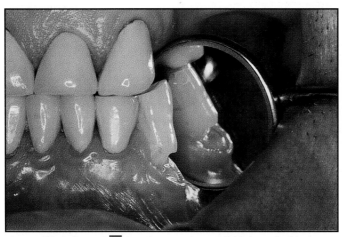

Fig. 7 Labial view of 3̄ showing 'V'-shaped labial cervical lesion

1 Flint S, Scully C. Orofacial age changes and related disease. *Dent Update* 1988; **15**: 337-342.

2 Smith B G N, Knight J K. An index for measuring the wear of teeth. *Br Dent J* 1984; **156**: 435-438.

3 Watson I B, Tulloch E N. Clinical assessment of cases of tooth surface loss. *Br Dent J* 1985; **159**: 144-148.

4 Bishop K A, Briggs P F A, Kelleher M G D. The aetiology and management of localized anterior tooth wear in the young adult. *Dent Update* 1994; **21**: 153-161.

5 Robb, N. *Epidemiological study of tooth wear.* London: University of London, 1991. PhD Thesis.

6 O'Brien M. *Childrens dental health in the United Kingdom.* London: HMSO, 1994.

7 Eccles J D. Tooth surface loss from abrasion, attrition and erosion. *Dent Update* 1982; **35**: 373-381.

8 Smith B G N. Some facets of toothwear. *Ann R Aust Coll Dent Surg* 1991; **11**: 37-51.

9 Shaw L, Smith A. Erosion in children: An increasing clinical problem? *Dent Update* 1994; **21**: 103-106.

10 Smith B G N, Knight J K. A comparison of patterns of tooth wear with aetiological factors. *Br Dent J* 1984; **157**: 16-19.

11 Mair L H. Wear in dentistry — current terminology. *J Dent* 1992; **20**: 140-144.

12 Jarvinen V K, Rytomaa I I, Heinonen, O P. Risk factors in dental erosion. *J Dent Res* 1991; **70**: 942-947.

13 Kelleher M, Bishop K. Personal communication, 1994.

Abrasion

Abrasion is caused by abnormal rubbing of tooth tissue or restoration by a non-dental object eg pipe-smoking, hair-grips etc.[11] However, the most common cause is probably incorrect or over vigorous toothbrushing[37]; although Smith and Knight[10] found that the occurrence of abrasion was infrequent compared with other types of TSL (fig. 7). Furthermore, the location of some 'abrasive' lesions cannot be explained by toothbrushing alone and other TSL factors such as erosion may contribute to the problem.[9,37] Recently, interest has grown in the role of occlusal stresses in the development of cervical 'abrasive' lesions and the term abfraction has been used to describe these.

Prevalence

It is generally accepted that the prevalence of TSL increases with age.[5,40–42] However, the exact prevalence is unclear, primarily because of differing assessment criteria.[42] Hugoson *et al.*,[39] for example, reported that 13–24% of surfaces showed evidence of occlusal wear. Other studies have observed that between 25% and 50% of subjects had evidence of TSL.[9] Some loss of tooth tissue is normal during a patients' lifetime as a result of 'wear and tear'. The loss is likely to be a problem only when the degree exceeds what would be considered 'normal' for a particular age. Studies which consider only 'pathological' TSL may, therefore, be more relevant to clinical dentistry. The tooth wear index (TWI)[2] attempted to achieve this by proposing maximum acceptable tooth tissue loss for each decade of life. Tooth surface loss in excess of these figures was considered 'pathological'. Using this index, between 4.5 and 5.7% of surfaces examined exhibited TSL.[2,5]

Although the actual prevalence of TSL is unclear, there is general agreement that the population, particularly the young, is experiencing increased exposure to elements which cause TSL.[4,5] The exact reason for this is unclear but the following factors may be implicated:

Body image

In the 1980s, fashion designers and image makers have promoted the concept that 'slimness' equates with 'attractive' or 'successful'. This concept is supported by role models who may have significantly influenced young people's perception of the 'ideal' body shape. In an attempt to control body weight patients may consume acidic foods such as fruit and diet drinks rather than high calorie alternatives. This struggle to achieve the 'ideal' body shape may also partly account for the increased prevalence of eating disorders.

Soft drink manufacturers

The soft drink industry is a multi-million pound business. Coca-Cola, for example, is the biggest brand label in the world with an estimated brand value of nearly $9,000 million. Marketing of soft drinks, traditionally, has been directed to the young adult by associating the beverages with peer group acceptability. More recently, the drinks have been promoted as 'healthy' and linked to high profile sportsmen and women. Consumption of acidic beverages following exercise may be more dangerous because of dehydration and a subsequent reduction in the buffering capacity of the saliva.

Refrigeration

Refrigeration has aided widespread accessibility to fruits, fruit-juices and soft drinks. It has allowed many fruits and vegetables to be available continually rather than when 'in season'. Consequently, diets can contain highly acidic foods and drinks all year round whereas previously many elements were restricted to particular times of the year.

Healthcare workers

Healthcare workers, such as doctors and dieticians, advocate that fresh fruit should be a component of a 'balanced' diet. These foods are, therefore, promoted as a 'healthy' option to 'harmful' alternatives. Patients are unlikely to be warned of the damage associated with acidic foods. Dentists may indirectly support this concept by advising their patients to avoid sugar. Patients may perceive that foods and drinks that do not contain sugar must therefore, be less damaging to their teeth. Dentists often suggest that patients should brush their teeth after exposure to foods and drinks containing sugar or acid, but such practices may accelerate TSL.[43]

Restorative materials

Dentists often use 'aesthetic' restorations, irrespective of whether the restoration is visible. Many of these materials have the potential to accelerate TSL, particularly if used on occluding surfaces in parafunctional patients (fig. 8).[44,45]

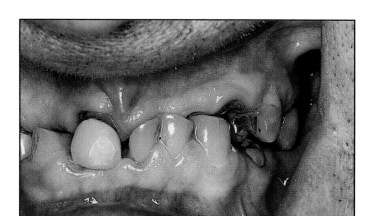

Fig. 8 Labial view of anterior teeth of a 60-year-old male with marked tooth surface loss affecting ⎿2⎿1⎿ caused by the abrasive porcelain palatal surface of ⎿1⎿

Clinical appearance of TSL

Although a 'classical' clinical appearance has been described for erosion, attrition and abrasion it is unlikely that the appearances described are a result of a single factor.[46] If dietary acid is applied to a tooth surface then the surface becomes frosty and white. However, the clinical 'erosive' lesion is smooth and polished.[37] Therefore attrition and/or abrasion is probably also present additionally. Even so, certain clinical features can indicate a dominant aetiological factor.

Teeth affected by erosion become rounded and lose their surface characteristics (figs. 4 and 5). Attrition, however, is associated with flattening of the cusp tips or incisal edges and localised facets on the occlusal or palatal surfaces (fig. 6). Following dentine exposure, the clinical appearance is determined by the relative contributions of the aetiological factors. If the TSL is primarily attritional then the dentine will wear at the same rate as the surrounding enamel. In this situation the shape of the facet will be determined by the movement of the opposing tooth. Traditionally it is suggested that when an erosive factor is present, 'cupping' or 'grooves' form in the dentine and the base of the defect is not in contact with the opposing tooth (fig. 4).[11] However, this may be an oversimplification of the changes that take place.

Cervical lesions caused by an abrasive tend to be angular and 'V'-shaped while erosion results in shallow, rounded lesions (fig. 7).

The clinical appearance of restorations may also indicate a possible major aetiological factor. Amalgam and composite restorations, for example, tend to be unaffected by erosive factors and remain 'proud' of the surrounding tooth tissue. However, both restorations show evidence of faceting if attrition is the major aetiological factor.[11]

Clinical problems

Aesthetics

Often a patient is only aware of TSL when there has been a deterioration in the appearance of the teeth. The earliest changes are because of the loss of enamel. This may cause an increase in tooth translucency, both interproximally and at the incisal edges.[46] Continued TSL may produce fractures of the enamel and shortening of the teeth.[47] The loss of enamel may also increase the visibility of the underlying dentine, producing a more yellow tooth colour.[4]

Conservation of tooth structure

The loss of tooth tissue is often substantial and the need to conserve remaining tooth structure is vital. This is particularly important in the young, where tooth tissue is at a premium because of the lack of secondary dentine. For this reason, 'adhesive' restorations should be considered before 'conventional' methods since the latter require further loss of tooth tissue.

Sensitivity and pain

Exposure of dentinal tubules and their subsequent bacterial colonisation can lead to both pulpal inflammation and sensitivity.[48] In younger patients with rapid erosion, this is further exacerbated by the lack of secondary dentine and large pulps. In extreme cases, pulpal exposure can occur, further complicating management (fig. 5).

Inter-occlusal space

Berry and Poole,[49] suggested that occlusal TSL is compensated by alveolar growth which maintains the occlusal vertical dimension (OVD). However, if the rate of loss is greater than the compensatory mechanism then the OVD is reduced. The effect of TSL on the occlusal vertical dimension is neither predictable nor uniform.

Patient compliance and expectations

Self-awareness and peer or social pressures may lead patients to refuse to comply with advice concerning the management of TSL. These

14 Rugg-Gunn A J, Hackett A F, Appleton D R, Jenkins G N, Eastoe J E. Relationship between dietary habits and caries increment assessed over two years in 405 English adolescent school children. *Arch Oral Biol* 1984; **29**: 983-987.

15 Eccles J D. Erosion affecting the palatal surfaces of upper anterior teeth in young people. *Br Dent J* 1982; **152**: 375-378.

16 Hellstrom, I. Oral complications in anorexia nervosa. *Scand J Dent Res* 1977; **85**: 71-86.

17 Giunta J L. Dental erosion resulting from chewable vitamin C tablets. *J Am Dent Assoc* 1983; **107**: 253-256.

18 Linkosalo E, Markkanen H. Dental erosions in relation to lactovegetarian diet. *Scand J Dent Res* 1985; **93**: 436-441.

19 Bartlett D W, Evans D F, Smith, B G N. Simultaneous oral and oesophageal pH measurement after a reflux provoking meal. *J Dent Res* 1994; Spec Issue Abst 70.

20 Jarvinen V, Meurman J H, Hyvarinen H *et al.* Dental erosion and upper gastrointestinal disorders. *Oral Surg Oral Med Oral Pathol* 1988; **65**: 298-303.

21 Howden G F. Erosion as the presenting symptom in hiatus hernia. *Br Dent J* 1971; **131**: 455-456

22 Rytomaa I, Jarvinen V, Heinonen, O P. Etiological factors in dental erosion. *J Dent Res* 1990; **69**: Spec. Issue. Abst 587.

23 Simmons M S, Thompson D C. Dental erosion secondary to ethanol-induced emesis. *Oral Surg Oral Med Oral Path* 1987; **64**: 731-713.

24 Smith B G N, Robb N D. Dental erosion in patients with chronic alcoholism. *J Dent* 1987; **17**: 219-221.

25 Bloem T J, McDowell G C, Lang B R *et al.* In vitro wear. Part II wear and abrasion of composite restorative materials. *J Prosthet Dent* 1988; **60**: 242-249.

26 Seymour R A. Dental pharmacology problems in the elderly. *Dent Update* 1988; **15**: 375-380.

27 Levine R.S. Saliva: 3. Xerostomia - aetiology and management. *Dent Update* 1989; **16**: 197-201.

28 Treasure J. Long-term management of eating disorders. *Int Rev Psych* 1991; **3**: 43-58.

29 Kidd E A M, Smith B G N. Toothwear histories: a sensitive issue. *Dent Update* 1989; **20**: 174-178.

30 Allen D N. Dental Erosion from Vomiting. *Br Dent J* 1969; **126**: 311-312.

31 Andrew F F H. Dental erosion due to anorexia nervosa with bulimia. *Br Dent J* 1982; **152**: 89-90.

32 Stege P, Visco-Dangler L, Rye L. Anorexia nervosa: review including oral & dental manifestations. *J Am Dent Assoc* 1982; **104**: 648-652.

33 Abrams R A, Ruff L C. Oral signs and symptoms in the diagnosis of bulimia. *J Am Dent Assoc* 1986; **113**: 761-764.

34 Gilmour A G, Beckett H A. The voluntary reflux phenomenon. *Br Dent J* 1993; **175**: 368-371.

35 Petersen P E, Gormsen C. Oral conditions among German battery factory workers. *Community Dent Oral Epidemiol* 1991; **19**: 104-106.

36 Centerwall B S, Armstrong C W, Funkerhouser L S, Elzay R. Erosion of dental enamel among competitive swimmers at a gas-chlorinated swimming pool. *Am J Epidemiol* 1986; **123**: 641-647.

37 Smith B G N. Toothwear: aetiology and diagnosis. *Dent Update* 1989; **16**: 204-212.

38 Krogh-Poulson W, Carlsen O R. *Bidfunktion/Bettfysiologi.* Denmark: Munksgaard, Kobenhavn. 1979, p269.

39 Dahl B L, Krogstad O, Karlsen K. An alternative treatment in cases with advanced localized attrition. *J Oral Rehabil* 1975; **2**: 209-214.

40 Hugoson A, Bergendal T, Ekfeldt A, Helkimo M. Prevalence and severity of incisal and occlusal tooth wear in an adult Swedish population. *Acta Odontol Scand* 1988; **46**: 255-265.

41 Ekfeldt A, Hugoson A, Bergendal T, Helkimo M. An individual tooth wear index and an analysis of factors correlated to incisal and occlusal wear in an adult Swedish population. *Acta Odontol Scand* 1990; **48**: 343-349.

42 Donachie M A. The dental health of the ageing population of Newcastle upon Tyne. Newcastle: University of Newcastle, 1992. MDS thesis .

43 Davis W B, Winter P J. The effect of abrasion on enamel and dentine after exposure to dietary acid. *Br Dent J* 1980; **148**: 253-256.

44 Jacobi R, Shillingburg H H T, Duncanson M G. A comparison of the abrasiveness of six ceramic surfaces and gold. *J Prosthet Dent* 1991; **66**: 303-309.

45 Ratledge D K, Smith B G N, Wilson, R F. The effect of restorative materials on the wear of human enamel. *J Prosthet Dent* 1994; **72**: 194-203.

46 Eccles J D, Jenkins W G. Dental erosion and diet. *J Dent* 1974; **2**: 153-159.

47 Eccles J D. Dental erosion of non industrial origin. A clinical survey and classification. *J Pros Dent* 1979; **42**: 649-653.

48 Brannstrom M. The cause of postrestorative sensitivity and its prevention. *J Endodont* 1986; **10**: 475-481.

49 Berry D C, Poole D F G. Attrition: possible mechanisms of compensation. *J Oral Rehabil* 1976; **3**: 201-206.

50 Kidd A M, Joyston-Bechal S. Essentials of dental caries: the disease and its management. Chapts 6 and 7. Bristol: Wright, 1987.

51 Bartlett D W, Smith B G N, Wilson, R F. Comparison of the effect of fluoride and non-fluoride toothpaste on tooth wear in vitro and the influence of enamel fluoride concentration and hardness of enamel. *Br Dent J* 1994; **176**: 346-348.

52 Gierdrys-Leeper E. Night guards and occlusal splints. *Dent Update* 1990; **17**: 325-329.

53 Kleier D J, Aragon S B, Averbach, R E. Dental management of the chronic vomiting patient. *J Am Dent Assoc* 1984; **108**: 618-621.

concerns may result in the rejection of a proposed restorative treatment plan: metal palatal restorations, for example, may be unacceptable because of 'grey-out'.[4] It is important that the implications of non-compliance and treatment alternatives are fully discussed with the patient.

Management

Immediate therapy

The aim of the immediate phase of therapy is to:

- Relieve sensitivity and pain
- Identify aetiological factors
- Protect remaining tooth tissue.

All aetiological factors for the TSL should be identified and eliminated although full compliance may be difficult. At the very least a 'damage limitation' policy should be initiated. This should involve identification, control and advice relating to the causative factors. Consideration should be given to the following:

- Diet analysis and counselling to control or reduce the effect of aetiological factors.[50]
- Advice to consume erosive beverages through a wide-bore straw and to swallow immediately and not 'swish' the drink around the mouth. Although teeth should not be brushed immediately following exposure to erosive factors, the exact 'safe' time period when oral hygiene can be carried out is unknown. This may reduce the risk of abrasive TSL.[9,43]
- Prescription of a neutral, sodium fluoride mouthrinse or gel for daily use to combat acid damage and control pulpal sensitivity.[51] Acidulated phosphate fluoride should be avoided because of its obvious acidity.
- Construction of a close fitting occlusal guard in those suspected of parafunctioning or where the aetiology is uncertain.[52] A guard may also be useful in bulimics to protect the teeth during periods of vomiting. Alkali, such as milk of magnesia, can be applied to the fitting surface of the guard to neutralise any acid pooling or alternatively a neutral fluoride gel placed in the appliance.[53] Appliances covering teeth must be used with extreme caution if there is a chance of acid being trapped beneath them.
- Direct application of glass ionomer and/or composite to sensitive areas.
- Consultation with the general medical practitioner regarding involuntary acidic reflux and/or psychiatrists to evaluate the patient's psychological status and background, especially in cases of bulimia nervosa.

Reassessment

Following immediate therapy, a period of time should elapse before a long-term treatment plan is considered allowing an evaluation of the patient's response to initial care. The reassessment should include whether the original aetiological factors are still present although this can be difficult to determine. Treatment needs can also be evaluated during this time and the patient's views and expectations considered.

Long-term management

The treatment planning options available are:

Review and monitoring

Providing the patient has no functional, occlusal, aesthetic or sensitivity problems following stabilisation then close monitoring of the situation is acceptable. This should involve the construction of accurate study casts: a set of casts should be given to the patient so that if there is a change in dentist, the records are available. Colour transparencies or photographs are also useful. A regular recall regime should be initiated and the patient instructed to return if they suspect any deterioration. If the rate of TSL is likely to jeopardise the tooth's long-term viability, then monitoring of the situation alone is unwise and restoration becomes necessary.

Restorative treatment

Restorative treatment is indicated when stabilisation techniques have failed to resolve the patient's dental problems. It is a widely-held view that restorative treatment in the presence of ongoing TSL is unwise. Nevertheless, there are occasions when control proves impossible and, to preserve the teeth, restoration becomes essential. The patients should be aware of both the advantages and disadvantages of any proposed treatment. Restoration should be based on the following principles:

- Protection and conservation of remaining tooth structure
- Resolution of pulpal sensitivity
- Improvement in aesthetics if necessary.

Conclusion

The paper has placed considerable emphasis on the aetiology of tooth surface loss as without an understanding of this, prevention and control are impossible. One of the major concerns in the United Kingdom is the increased incidence of TSL caused by acid erosion. Many of the reasons for this are dietary but others relate to regurgitation of acid. The next article in this series will discuss eating disorders in detail and the management of patients who are affected by this seemingly increasingly common condition.

This article is based on a presentation at The Medical Society of London on 5 October 1994 as part of the Alpha Omega lecture programme.

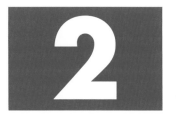

2 Eating disorders and the dentist

A. Milosevic[1]

The first article in this series provided an overview of tooth surface loss. It included a preliminary discussion of involuntary and voluntary regurgitation of gastric acid. The second article is devoted to the subject of eating disorders, the regurgitation of gastric acid and how patients affected by these conditions may present to the dentist. The likelihood that a general dental practitioner will have an eating disordered subject on their patient list is quite high. Furthermore, anorexia occurs in upper and middle class families while bulimia presents across all social classes.[1] It is, therefore, desirable that dentists have some understanding of the eating disorders and their manifestations.

Definitions, diagnostic criteria and epidemiology

Anorexia nervosa
Anorexia may be defined as: 'aversion to food resulting from a complex interaction between biological, social, individual and family factors leading to severe weight loss'. The diagnostic criteria change as more is understood about its psychopathology, but currently there are two subtypes: the 'restricting' and the 'binge/purge'. The distinction between the two is based on whether the person regularly engages in binge eating or purging behaviour (ie self-induced vomiting, strenuous exercise or misuse of laxatives, diuretics or enemas).

The incidence is 7 per 100,000 with around 4,000 new cases per annum in the UK and a prevalence ranging from 0.1 to 1% of young females.[1]

Bulimia nervosa
Bulimia is more common than anorexia with an incidence of between 8.6 and 14 per 100,000 of the total population, with about 1 to 2% of adolescent girls and young women affected by the disorder.[1,2] As with anorexia, the American Psychiatric Association and WHO diagnostic criteria differ, but over-eating followed by inappropriate compensatory behaviour are key features of bulimia. Eating disorders occur predominately in young females (F:M ratio of 10:1) with 16 years being the average age of presentation for anorexia and a later presentational age of 25 for bulimia nervosa.[1] Uni- and multi-impulsive bulimia nervosa have been described. In addition to binge

eating and purging, the latter may engage in alcohol or drug abuse, shoplifting, promiscuity and aberrant sexual practices. In general, anorexics are more than 15% below ideal body weight whereas bulimics are within 10% of ideal weight or can be overweight. An anorexic will look thin: the bulimic is less readily identifiable from their outward appearance.

Risk factors, psychological and medical complications of eating disorders
The fashion and media industries have conceptualised the 'ideal' modern female form as slim, either in response to some vague societal norm or have promoted this form themselves. The consequent pressure to control weight has led to an over-concern with body image and dieting particularly in susceptible females and even in healthy children. The susceptibilities or risk factors associated with eating disorders are shown in Table 1.

Studies on twins show that anorectic traits and the full syndrome have a genetic component.[3,4] Early menarche, a feature of childhood obesity, which in turn increases the risk of early dieting are high risks for developing bulimia. Family dysfunction, however, may not be contributory in anorexia, although families with an anorectic have been described as high achieving, over-protective and conflict avoiding. Inter-personal relationships within the families of a bulimia sufferer seem to have greater significance in its aetiology and maintenance. Childhood sexual and physical abuse, parental overexpectations coupled with hypercriticism, parental indifference and emotional immaturity all frequently appear in the bulimic family background. Broadly, bulimics tend to be more extrovert whereas anorexics are characterised as introverted. Low self esteem and perfectionism are common personality traits in both conditions. Undoubtedly dieting precedes an eating disorder. Should target weight or shape

Table 1 Risk factors associated with eating disorders

Biological:	Fat metabolism, abnormal 5HT function
Demographic:	Female, social class
Dieting	
Familial:	Family dysfunction, positive family history
Genetic	
Occupational:	Models, dancers, athletes
Psychological:	Stress, low self esteem, perfectionism, depression

Dentists are likely to encounter patients who have eating disorders. The paper explains the various types and considers both the risk factors, and the psychological and medical complications. The effect on oral health and the principles of dental management are outlined. Dentists have an important part to play in the overall care of these patients.

[1]*Lecturer in Restorative Dentistry, Department of Clinical Dental Sciences, The University of Liverpool, Liverpool L69 3BX*

tooth surface loss

Table 2 Medical problems of eating disorders

System	Starvation	Purging/vomiting
Blood	Anaemia Thrombocytopenia Leucopenia	
Cardiovascular	Bradycardia	Arrythmias and sudden death
	Hypotension	Cardiac failure ECG abnormalities
CNS	Cerebral changes Cognitive damage	Epileptic fits Tetany
Endocrine	Ovarian changes Ammenorhoea Reduced oestrogen and progesterone Increased cortisol and growth hormone Diabetes insipidus	
Gastro-intestinal	Delayed gastric emptying and poor motility Malabsorption	Oesophageal ulcers Constipation/diarrhoea
Liver	Raised enzymes Fatty infiltration	
Musculo-skeletal	Osteoporosis Pathological fractures	Myopathy
Renal	Reduced glomerular filtration	Electrolyte abnormalities: reduced Na and K increased P and Mg
Skin/hair	Loss of head hair Lanugo	

not be achieved from dieting, the resultant feelings of failure or depression tip the individual into bulimia. This furthers the sense of guilt and low self esteem, compounding the inadequacy felt by many sufferers.

The medical complications are wide ranging and mainly attributable to nutritional deficiencies and weight control practices (Table 2).

The physical consequences of anorexia

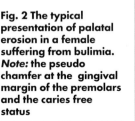

Fig. 1 Callus on the back of the hand (Russell's sign) in a 37-year-old male with a history of bulimia nervosa of 20 years' duration

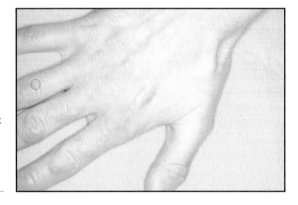

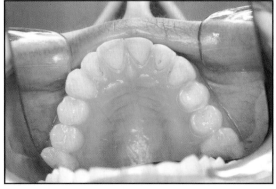

Fig. 2 The typical presentation of palatal erosion in a female suffering from bulimia. *Note:* the pseudo chamfer at the gingival margin of the premolars and the caries free status

include emaciation, hypotension, bradycardia, cyanosis and menstrual irregularities coupled with ovarian changes. Serum oestrogen is low. Coping with puberty, sexual development and initial heterosexual relationships places great emotional stress on adolescents which for some is resolved by avoiding weight gain through strict dietary control and disordered eating. The consequent stunting of growth, amennorhoea and prepubetal regression become self-fulfilling and help maintain the disorder.

The median duration of these illnesses is up to 6 years with significant mortality (4–20%) from medical complications and suicide in anorexia nervosa.[1] Bulimia seems to have a better outcome with death a rare consequence (0.3%).[2]

Callus formation on the back of the hand and fingers from putting the hand in the mouth to induce vomiting can be present and is called Russell's sign (Fig. 1).

Oro-dental effects of the eating disorders

Erosion
Holst and Lange (1939) coined the term 'perimylolysis' to describe the distribution of erosion on the upper palatal surfaces secondary to vomiting, reflux and regurgitation.[5] They cited a 1929 thesis by Fleury as the source for the term 'mylolysis' which alluded to the slow destruction of coronal tooth tissue. Neither term is useful since they are not specific descriptors for the distribution of intrinsic erosion: extrinsic erosion has a similar intra-oral presentation (Fig. 2).[6]

The impact of eating disorders upon oral health was initially reported by Hellstrom (1977)[7] and Hurst *et al.* (1977).[8] Since then there have been dozens of case reports and reviews.[9–12] The original publications found that the severity and distribution of dental erosion differed according to whether or not the subjects induced vomiting.[7,8] In general, self-induced vomiting (SIV) resulted in an increased frequency of erosion on palatal surfaces but both research groups noted that the diet of their subjects included significant quantities of low pH beverages and fresh fruit. The latter was eaten to induce diarrhoea. A third of both the anorexics and bulimics sampled by Roberts and Li were reported to suffer with erosion despite the observation that only 65% of the anorexics vomited compared to all the bulimics.[13] The strength of association between vomiting and erosive toothwear was not assessed until more recently. The frequency, duration and total number of vomiting episodes (frequency ↔ duration) were not linearly associated with erosion[14] and similarly no difference in the level of erosion was found between those who vomited more or less frequently.[15] Both studies, however, reported an increased frequency of erosion in subjects with SIV and therefore some other factor(s) must be involved in determining whether or not erosion occurs.

The distribution of erosion

Mean palatal and upper anterior buccal (labial) toothwear scores were significantly greater in vomiting anorexics and bulimics compared with abstaining anorexics and controls.[15] A further result from the same study was that both the abstaining and vomiting anorexics exhibited more lower posterior wear on buccal and occlusal surfaces than controls.[15] Why the non-vomiting abstainers exhibit buccal and occlusal toothwear is unclear although Scheutzel reported that buccal and/or labial erosion occurred in those bulimics who drank 'larger quantities of acidic foods'.[16] She believed that SIV initially affected the palatal and occlusal surfaces whereas extrinsic acids resulted in vestibular erosions. According to Scheutzel, however, regular vomiting for 5 years or more could also affect facial surfaces. Milosevic and Slade found that erosion was more likely after 1100 vomiting episodes and that the intra-oral distribution was primarily upper palatal, occlusal and cervical.[14] The widely held belief that intrinsic (gastric) acid results in palatally eroded sites and extrinsic (dietary) acids lead to labial erosion remains controversial. Jarvinen et al. reported that the cause of erosion could not be reliably determined from its location although palatal erosion was slightly more frequent in the gastric aetiology group compared with the dietary group.[6]

Caries

Whether the caries experience of eating disordered individuals is greater than the normal population remains unclear. Caries experience was no different between vomiters and non-vomiters in Hellstrom's study[7] while Hurst et al.[8] reported non-vomiters to have less caries experience. Neither of these studies had controls, or used recognised indices and the data were not statistically analysed. Similar results from three continents found no difference in the caries experience between anorexics, bulimics and controls.[14,17,18] These findings were not corroborated by Philipp et al. who reported lower mean DMFT in disordered eating groups compared with their control group[19] while Altshuler reported greater decay in bulimia nervosa.[20] This was corroborated by Rytomaa et al. who reported that their bulimic sample exhibited more proximal and bucco-lingual caries than age, sex and education matched controls.[21] Perfectionist tendencies or obsessional-compulsive traits are common in anorexics and bulimics which may manifest dentally with good oral hygiene.[22] Qualitative rather than quantitative differences, such as the cariogenicity of the oral flora, may occur and be dependent upon vomiting parameters.

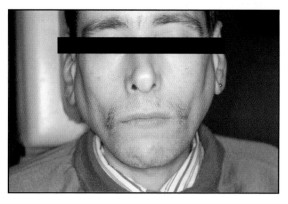

Fig. 3 Bilateral parotid enlargement; this is episodic

Saliva

The salivary functions of lubrication and neutralisation of intra-oral acids particularly after SIV are probably important in eating disorders. Salivary flow increases dramatically prior to vomiting because the medullary centre that controls vomiting is connected to salivary nuclei.[23] The nausea provoked by oesophageal and stomach distension after binge eating further stimulates salivation.[24] With respect to SIV, therefore, stimulated salivary flow should be of more consequence. According to Hellstrom,[7] resting salivary flow was poor although stimulated flow rates were within the normal range. Normal stimulated flow was reported in non-vomiting restricting anorexics and bulimics by Touyz et al.[18] while Milosevic and Dawson found significantly lower rates in vomiting bulimics with and without erosion compared with controls.[25] The latter study also assessed bicarbonate concentration and viscosity. It discovered reduced bicarbonate in both bulimic groups but increased salivary viscosity in the bulimics with erosion. The low bicarbonate will act as a co-factor in erosion cases but does not fully explain why some bulimics do not exhibit erosion despite the poor buffer capacity. Stimulated and unstimulated salivary concentrations of potassium, chloride, calcium, urea nitrogen and albumin were reported to be within normal values.[26]

Changes in salivary secretion, may be secondary to structural change within the gland. Episodic benign parotid enlargement has been described in bulimics by several workers[27–30] and is shown in figure 3. Gland biopsy was performed in one case with no apparent abnormality.[27] It should be noted, however, that other than at its site, the biopsy gives no information on the rest of the structure.

It seems that the metabolic disturbances in eating disorders do not necessarily result in altered salivary characteristics.

Microbiology

Very few studies have analysed the oral microbial flora in eating disordered subjects. A repeatedly low intra-oral pH from SIV could theoretically manifest as a change in normal flora to a more aciduric type. *Streptococcus*

1 Hugo P J, Lacey J H. Eating disorders — diagnosis and management. *Primary Care Psych* 1996; **2**: 87-100.
2 Schmidt U, Treasure J. Eating disorders and the dental practitioner. *Eur J Prosthodont Rest Dent* 1997; **5**: 161-167.
3 Rutherford J, McGuffin P, Katz R J, Murray R M. Genetic influences on eating attitudes in a normal female twin population. *Psychol Med* 1993; **23**: 425-436.
4 Strober M, Lampert C, Morrell W, Burroughs J, Jacobs C. A controlled family study of anorexia nervosa: evidence of familial aggregation and lack of shared transmission with affective disorders. *Int J Eating Disorders* 1990; **9**: 239-253.
5 Holst J J, Lange F. Perimylolysis. A contribution towards the genesis of tooth wasting from non-mechanical causes. *Acta Odontol Scand* 1939; **1**: 36-47.
6 Jarvinen V, Rytomaa I, Meurmann J H. Location of dental erosion in a referred population. *Caries Res* 1992; **26**: 391-396.
7 Hellstrom I. Oral complications in anorexia nervosa. *Scand J Dent Res* 1977; **85**: 71-86.
8 Hurst P S, Lacey J H, Crisp A H. Teeth, vomiting and diet: a study of

the dental characteristics of seventeen anorexia nervosa patients. *Postgrad Med J* 1977; **53**: 298-305.

9 Stege P, Visco-Dangler L, Rye L. Anorexia nervosa: review including oral and dental manifestations. *J Am Dent Assoc* 1982; **104**: 648-652.

10 Wolcott R B, Yager J, Gordon G. Dental sequelae to the binge purge syndrome (bulimia): report of cases. *J Am Dent Assoc* 1984; **109**: 723-725.

11 Burke F J T, Bell T J, Ismail N, Hartley P. Bulimia: implications for the practising dentist. *Br Dent J* 1996; **180**: 421-426.

12 Robb N D, Smith B G N. Anorexia and bulimia nervosa (the eating disorders): conditions of interest to the dental practitioner. *J Dent* 1996; **24**: 7-16

13 Roberts M W, Li S-H. Oral findings in anorexia nervosa and bulimia nervosa: a study of 47 cases. *J Am Dent Assoc* 1987; **115**: 407-410.

14 Milosevic A, Slade P D. The orodental status of anorexics and bulimics. *Br Dent J* 1989; **167**: 66-70.

15 Robb N D, Smith B G N, Geidrys-Leeper E. The distribution of erosion in the dentitions of patients with eating disorders. *Br Dent J* 1995; **178**: 171-175.

16 Scheutzel P. Etiology of dental erosion — intrinsic factors. *Eur J Oral Sci* 1996; **104**: 178-190.

17 Jones R R H, Cleaton-Jones P. Depth and area of dental erosions and dental caries in bulimic women. *J Dent Res* 1989; **68**: 1275-1278.

18 Touyz S W, Liew V P, Tseng P, Frisken K, Williams H, Beumont P J V. Oral and dental complications in dieting disorders. *Int J Eating Disord* 1993; **18**: 341-348.

19 Philipp E, Willershausen-Zonnchen B, Hamm G, Pirke K-M. Oral and dental characteristics in bulimic and anorectic patients. *Int J Eating Disord* 1991; **10**: 423-431.

20 Altshuler B D, Dechow P C, Waller D A, Hardy B W. An investigation of the oral pathologies occurring in bulimia nervosa *Int J Eating Disord* 1990; **9**: 191-199.

21 Rytmaa I, Jarvinen V, Kanerva R, Heinonen O P. Bulimia and tooth erosion. *Acta Odontol Scand* 1998; **56**: 36-40.

22 Terry-Short L A, Glynn Owens R, Slade P D, Dewey M E. Positive and negative perfectionism. *Person Individ Diff* 1995; **18**: 663-668.

23 Edgar W M. Saliva: Its secretion, composition and functions. *Br Dent J* 1992; **172**: 305-312.

24 Jenkins G N. In: *The physiology and biochemistry of the mouth.* 4th ed. Oxford: Blackwell Scientific Publications, 1978.

25 Milosevic A, Dawson L J. Salivary factors in vomiting bulimics with and without pathological tooth wear. *Caries Res* 1996; **30**: 361-366.

26 Tylenda C A, Roberts M W, Elin R J, Li S-H, Altemus M. Bulimia nervosa: its effect on salivary chemistry. *J Am Dent Assoc* 1991; **122**: 37-41.

27 Levin P A, Falko J M, Dixon K, Gallup E M, Saunders W. Benign parotid enlargement in bulimia. *Ann*

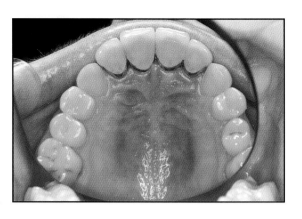

Fig. 4 A bizarre palatal haematoma in this 30-year-old female bulimic was of no concern to the patient. Note again the low caries activity

mutans and Lactobacillus counts were no different between anorexics, bulimics and controls although the authors do not state whether they assessed plaque or saliva.[18] Salivary *S sobrinus* levels were significantly higher in bulimics but neither *S mutans*, *Lactobacilli* nor yeast were different.[31] A follow-up fluoxetine and placebo-based study reported a decrease in the *S sobrinus* salivary count during 16 weeks in bulimics on the medication.[32] The authors felt that salivary levels of these organisms could act as a marker of patient compliance with antibulimic therapy. Further research in this area would be of value.

Periodontal disease

The evidence on periodontal status is conflicting. The earlier reports without controls found unremarkable plaque and gingival levels and no differences between anorexics and bulimics.[7,8] Gingival index scores were not statistically different between groups of anorexics, bulimics and controls.[13,14,20] Philipp *et al.* reported greater sulcus bleeding in their control group,[19] whereas Touyz *et al.* found fewer bleeding sites in their controls.[18] Loss of attachment was no greater among eating disordered subjects.[18,20]

Soft tissue lesions

Angular cheilitis, candidosis, glossitis and oral mucosal ulceration are possible sequelae to nutritional deficiencies. A peculiar intra-oral presentation may raise suspicions in the dentist's mind that something odd is happening. The large palatal haematoma, shown in figure 4, was painfree and an incidental finding in a 26-year-old female bulimic. A lingual abscess of dental origin was reported in an anorexic with possible secondary immuno-deficiency as a predisposing factor.[33] Despite the potential chronic irritation to the mucosa from long term vomiting, contrary to one anecdote,[34] there has not been any report of malignant change associated with SIV.

Dental management

The dentist can provide general advice and routine through to complex treatment for the severely eroded dentition. The dental care demanded by the eating disordered individual is perhaps more specific than for other patients but not necessarily specialised. The approach should be non-judgmental and sympathetic.[35] Although the dentist might suspect vomiting as the cause of the erosion, the eating disordered patient will not readily admit to such behaviour because they can be highly secretive and embarrassed by it.

The timing of restorative intervention for eroded teeth is controversial. Caries and periodontal disease should be managed as usual but should the dentist wait for the vomiting to be controlled before restoring the worn surfaces? There is no definite contra-indication to restoring eroded surfaces other than the continued acid dissolution of tooth substance from around the restoration should the vomiting continue. While providing initial therapy and fillings, the toothwear can be monitored with study casts and photographs, and the patient will hopefully gain confidence in the dentist. The patient may then be more inclined to discuss their disordered eating and purging. Motivation to reduce the frequency of SIV is therefore more likely once the dentist can openly relate the progress of dental erosion with the vomiting. Pain relief, reduced dentine sensitivity and improved appearance are further factors which will motivate the patient. The dentist can make several recommendations to the anorexic and bulimic (Table 3). Some of this is general advice for patients with erosion while certain points are aimed at the eating disordered patient.

Toothbrushing after vomiting is generally regarded as inadvisable because the softened, demineralised surface is more susceptible to toothbrush abrasion. Two research groups assessed post vomiting oral hygiene practices with the degree of toothwear and independently found that the wear was no worse in eating disordered subjects who brushed immediately after vomiting.[15,36]

The treatment plan will be dependent on several parameters and it would be impossible to cover all eventualities within the scope of this paper. Some broad aspects of examination and treatment can be discussed. The

Table 3 Recommendations to minimise dental problems in eating disorders

Raise awareness of sources of acid in the diet, thus:
- Reduce intake of acidic drinks, drink alternatives (low calorie beverages are usually consumed but they still have erosive potential)
- Reduce consumption of fresh fruit especially citrus fruit
- Alcohol in various guises eg white wine, mixers, cider, alcopops

Post-vomiting methods of increasing pH and improving oral milieu:
- After self-induced (SIV) vomiting chew gum, rinse mouth with water or milk
- Rinsing with an antacid preparation
- Gentle toothbrushing with a small amount of desensitising or bicarbonate toothpaste after SIV may be safe

Check that any medication does not provoke dry mouth or nausea

For salivary hypofunction/dry mouth:
- Prescribe neutral artificial saliva or sialogogue pastilles eg Saliva Orthana spray and lozenges (Nycomed UK Ltd, Birmingham); Salivix pastilles (Thames Laboratories Ltd, Wrexham)

interocclusal space is examined in the intercuspal position (ICP). Even a space of less than 1 mm is amenable to restoration with composite bonded to dentine. In the author's opinion any eroded and sclerosed dentine should be over etched (20–30s) in order to enhance opening of dentinal tubules and intratubular formation of resin tags.[37] Furthermore, the intertubular or hybrid zone will be better wetted for so-called wet bonding should some outflow of pulpal fluid occur. Composite restoratives are not acid soluble and thus preferable to polyalkenoate (glass ionomer) materials which have no place in the restoration of teeth when SIV is still a continuing problem. Adhesive dentistry has advantages over conventional forms of treatment in that it is reversible and the latest generation of dentine bonding agents are durable. Apart from bonding composite to eroded surfaces, many workers have described bonding porcelain[38] and metal veneers,[39] metal onlays,[40] a combination 'double veneer',[41] or resin (dentine) bonded crowns.[42] Many of these alternatives are covered in detail later in the series. Part 5 discusses the adhesive clinical techniques which can be used under these circumstances. The conservative nature of adhesive restorations makes them attractive for erosive TSL. They permit early restorative intervention when this is considered essential to protect the tooth structure that remains, while avoiding many of the problems inherent in conventional crowns. Space requirements are still minimal when using these adhesive techniques. However, after examining in ICP, the dentist should check the amount of slide from retruded axis position to ICP and see if any distal mandibular repositioning could gain valuable anterior space. Should dentoalveolar compensation have occurred, such that there is no interocclusal space in the anterior region, then a Dahl appliance can be considered.[43]

The dentist should liaise with the medical practitioner. Medication, usually antidepressants for bulimia, may influence salivary flow. The progress of behavioural therapy can help the dentist better plan the stages of dental treatment. Greater emphasis is currently placed on management, education and counselling within the primary care setting.[44] Denial and shame are strong features of eating disorders such that many sufferers attempt to conceal problems or present with other symptoms.[1] Unexplained weight loss, abdominal and gynaecological problems, sore throat from recurrent vomiting, poor sleep, lethargy and fatigue should alert primary care staff to possible disordered eating habits. Less severe cases of anorexia are amenable to long term out-patient psychotherapy or counselling coupled with medical monitoring. In-patient treatment for more advanced cases of anorexia and the mutli-impulsive bulimic involves nutritional provision and psychotherapy. Details of regional self-help network contacts are available from: The Eating Disorders Association, 1st Floor, Wensum House, 103 Prince of Wales Road, Norwich NR1 1DW, *Tel:* 01603 621414.

There is a better outcome for bulimia with recovery in up to 80% but only 50% of anorexia nervosa sufferers recover weight and normal menstrual patterns.[45]

Conclusion
Patients whose teeth have been damaged as a consequence of an eating disorder are most likely to present first to the dentist in general practice. This paper has helped clarify the nature of the condition, and the medical and dental pictures on patients' presentation. The dentist may in some cases be in a position to assist in making the initial diagnosis and can influence progress of the medical and psychological management by providing support and dental care.

Int Med 1980; **93**: 827-829.
28 Hasler J F. Parotid enlargement: A presenting sign in anorexia nervosa. *Oral Surg Oral Med Oral Pathol* 1982; **53**: 567-573.
29 Burke C. Bulimia and parotid enlargement — case report and treatment. *J Otolaryngol* 1986; **15**: 49-51.
30 Taylor V E, Sneddon J. Bilateral facial swelling in bulimia. Br Dent J 1987; **163**: 115-117.
31 Bretz W A, Krahn D D, Drewnowski A, Loesche W J. Salivary levels of putative cariogenic organisms in patients with eating disorders. *Oral Microbiol Immunol* 1989; **4**: 230-232.
32 Bretz W A, Krahn D D, Drury M, Schork N, Loesche W J. Effects of fluoxetine on the oral environment of bulimics. *Oral Microbiol Immunol* 1993; **8**: 62-64.
33 Keith O, Flint S, Scully C. Lingual abscess in a patient with anorexia nervosa. Br Dent J 1989; **167**: 71-72.
34 Brady W F. The anorexia nervosa syndrome. *Oral Med Oral Surg Oral Pathol* 1980; **50**: 509-516.
35 Kidd E A M, Smith B G N. Toothwear histories. A sensitive issue. *Dent Update* 1993; **20**: 1174-1178.
36 Milosevic A, Brodie D A, Slade P D. Dental erosion, oral hygiene, and nutrition in eating disorders. *Int J Eat Disord* 1997; **21**: 195-199.
37 Van Meerbeek B, Braem M, Lambrechts P, Vanherle G. Morphological characterisation of the interface between resin and sclerotic dentine. *J Dent* 1994; **22**: 141-146.
38 Milosevic A. The use of porcelain veneers to restore palatal tooth surface loss. *Rest Dent* 1990; **6**: 15-18.
39 Darbar U R. The treatment of palatal erosive wear by using oxidised gold veneers: A case report. *Quintessence Int* 1994; **25**: 195-197.
40 Crawford P J M, Aboush Y E Y. The use of adhesively retained gold onlays in the management of dental erosion in a child: a 4-year case report. Br Dent J 1993; **175**: 414-416.
41 Bishop K, Bell M, Briggs P, Kelleher M. Restoration of a worn dentition using a double-veneer technique. Br Dent J 1996; **180**: 26-29.
42 Milosevic A, Jones C. Use of resin-bonded ceramic crowns in a bulimic patient with severe tooth erosion. *Quintessence Int* 1996; **27**: 123-127.
43 Dahl B L, Krogstad O, Karlsen K. An alternative treatment in cases with advanced localized attrition. *J Oral Rehabil* 1975; **2**: 209-214.
44 The Royal College of Psychiatrists. *Eating Disorders Council Report CR14: 1992.* London: The Royal College of Psychiatrists.
45 Steinhausen H-CH, Rauss-Mason C, Seidel R. Follow-up studies of anorexia nervosa: a review of four decades of outcome research. *Psychol Med* 1991; **21**: 447-454.

3 Occlusion and splint therapy

N. J. Capp[1]

The first two articles in the series concentrated on the aetiology and presentation of tooth surface loss. This paper begins to look at its consequences. Tooth wear can be considered pathological if the degree of wear exceeds the level expected at any particular age. Tooth surface loss affecting the functional surfaces creates difficulties for the restorative dentist and may affect the stability of the occlusion. The first part of this article discusses the importance of occlusal stability and the possible consequences when it is lost. The second part is devoted to the role of occlusal appliances in protecting teeth from wear and in some aspects of the pre-restorative management of tooth surface loss.

The occlusion

Most functional (chewing) and parafunctional (bruxing and clenching) movements of the mandible take place around the intercuspal position (ICP). This is defined as the mandibular position in which maximum intercuspation of the teeth occurs. Functional movements result in brief contacts between maxillary and mandibular teeth, usually toward the end of the masticatory cycle. However, parafunctional activity may produce prolonged periods of forceful tooth contact.

In 90% of the population maximum intercuspation occurs slightly forward from the retruded position of the mandible to the maxilla. However, contact between opposing teeth and the resultant proprioceptive response guides the mandible repeatedly into the habitual ICP, wherever it may be.

Should a patient exhibit parafunctional activity, it becomes increasingly important that there are enough opposing posterior teeth to provide stable ICP contacts, so that the forces produced during parafunction are distributed over a wide area and in the most favourable direction.

Stable ICP contacts are provided by natural or restored surfaces which have appropriately steep cuspal anatomy (fig. 1). Contact either between the tips of supporting cusps and opposing fossae, or three points surrounding each supporting cusp tip and the ridges surrounding the opposing fossa (tripodisation), provide stable ICP contacts which direct occlusal forces axially.

They will also, in conjunction with the proximal contacts of adjacent teeth, stabilise the positions of individual teeth and also of the mandible in ICP. If ICP contacts are unstable, tilting and tipping of teeth are more likely particularly in the absence of an intact arch. This will cause further loss of stable ICP contacts and increase the likelihood of interferences occurring between the posterior teeth during lateral and protrusive movements.

In order to reduce the potentially harmful lateral forces produced by bruxing on interferences between posterior teeth, it is desirable for a patient to possess adequate anterior guidance. Contact between opposing teeth, preferably the canines in lateral excursion and the central incisors in protrusion, discludes the posterior teeth as soon as the mandible moves from ICP (fig. 1). This occlusal scheme most importantly reduces the number of tooth contacts occurring outside ICP. There is some evidence that this alters the proprioceptive feedback to the central nervous system which in turn reduces the level of activity in the masticatory muscles,[1,2] although this view is hard to support on scientific grounds. However, in simple practical terms it is very much easier to make restorations in the presence of an adequately steep, immediate disclusion, provided by a small number of teeth near the front of the mouth.[3]

How may occlusal stability be maintained or lost?

Most restorations are made to conform to a patient's existing ICP. For this to be an appropriate form of treatment ICP must be stable and the occlusal anatomy of all restorations must be carefully shaped to reproduce correct contacts. In addition, the restorative materials used should be easy to manipulate to produce the necessary occlusal contacts, and exhibit similar wear characteristics to enamel or to opposing restorations. This will reduce the chance of differential wear and increase the likelihood of stable contacts being maintained long-term. Gold (fig. 2) is still the most suitable material based upon these criteria, while amalgam remains the plastic material of choice for posterior teeth. The use of composite resin (direct or indirect) or occlusal porcelain to restore large areas of multiple occlusal surfaces should be avoided in patients prone to parafunction and those with restricted anterior guidance. The difficulty in providing stable contacts and the surface hardness of these

**Control of occlusal contacts is important to the success of restorative dentistry. Tooth surface loss can contribute to a loss of stability in the occlusion.
An occlusal splint is often part of pre-restorative management and can also have a valuable role in protecting both teeth and restorations from excessive loads and further wear.**

[1]*Honorary Senior Research Fellow, Eastman Dental Institute for Oral Healthcare Sciences, University of London, 256 Gray's Inn Road, London WC1X 8LD and Specialist in Restorative Dentistry, 35 Harley Street, London W1N 1HA*

tooth surface loss

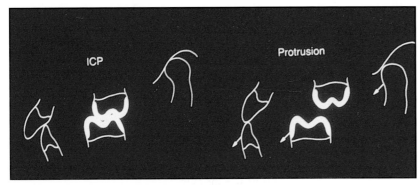

Fig. 1 Restorations with adequately steep cusps provide occlusal stability in ICP while discluding the lateral and protrusive movements

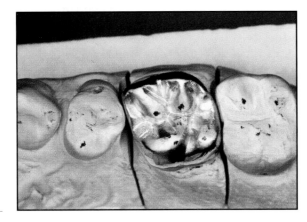

Fig. 2 Gold still provides the best means of restoring occlusal stability

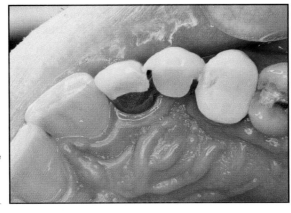

Fig. 3 A 3-unit fixed prosthesis with inadequate occlusal form and inappropriate choice of materials for the articulating surfaces

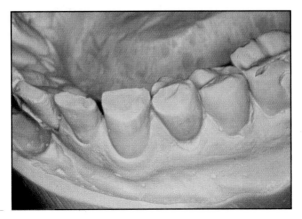

Fig. 4 Tooth surface loss because of the abrasive effect of the porcelain guidance surfaces on opposing teeth

materials may result in increased tooth surface loss in the opposing arch (fig. 3, 4). The careful use of occlusal porcelain and composite resin is less harmful in individuals who possess immediate disclusion of their posterior teeth and do not parafunction.

Loss of stable contacts may also occur because of tooth surface loss caused by acid erosion or parafunction between unrestored or similarly restored surfaces. Loss of cusp height and definition, broadening areas of ICP contact, combined with a shallowing of the anterior guidance, reduces stability and increases the chances of interferences in lateral or protrusive movements, causing increased and less favourable stress distribution in the teeth affected.

Loss of occlusal stability may result in the repeated fracture of restorations and teeth, increased mobility and drifting, particularly of the upper anterior segment. Traditionally, it has also been held to potentially have other long-term effects on the structure and function of the temporomandibular joints,[4,5] although such assertions are increasingly open to question. In the presence of any of these signs of loss of occlusal stability, it sometimes becomes necessary to reorganise the patient's occlusion creating a new and stable ICP at the retruded position of the mandible. There is little reason to choose the retruded position other than because of 'prosthetic convenience'. In the absence of a stable ICP, the retruded position is the only relationship of mandible to maxilla which can be repeatedly and consistently recorded and has been shown to be physiologically acceptable. It is also the maxillo-mandibular relationship to which the mandible will return when not prevented from doing so by interfering tooth contacts. It may therefore be used as the reference position in which the new restorations will intercuspate when re-organising the occlusion.

The rationale and indications for occlusal splints

An occlusal splint is a removable appliance covering some or all of the occlusal surfaces of the teeth in either the maxillary or mandibular arches. The ideal occlusal splint is made from laboratory-processed acrylic resin which should cover the occlusal surfaces of all the teeth in one arch. It should provide even simultaneous contacts on closure on the retruded axis with all opposing teeth and anterior guidance causing immediate disclusion of the posterior teeth and splint surface outside ICP.

The splint provides the patient with an ideal occlusion with posterior stability and anterior guidance. It will disrupt the habitual path of closure into ICP by separating the teeth and removing the guiding effect of the cuspal inclines. It causes an immediate and pronounced relaxation in the masticatory muscles,[6] which will eventually result in the mandible repositioning and closing in the retruded position uninterfered with by the teeth.

In order to achieve this muscle relaxation and mandibular repositioning the occlusal surface of the splint is flat and without indentations so as not to hold or guide the mandible into any predetermined position. The only exception to this is the area lateral to the canine and anterior to the incisor ICP contacts which is gently ramped to provide anterior guidance. To achieve muscle relaxation and repositioning of the mandible, the splint ideally must be worn continuously, failure to do so will result in an increase in masticatory muscle activity.[7,8] As the mandible repositions it is necessary to adjust the splint frequently to maintain even contact and disclusion.[9] However, continuous wear is often not compatible with the patient's daily activities. Wear at night and also if possible in the evenings will achieve the same result but more slowly.

Uses of splints
The use of an appropriate occlusal splint may be indicated in the following circumstances:

Prevention of tooth surface loss
Patients who are prone to nocturnal bruxism should routinely wear occlusal splints at night. The splint may reduce their parafunctional activity while it is being worn but as soon as it is removed masticatory muscle activity will resume its increased levels.[6] Whether or not bruxing is continuing can be monitored by observing wear facets created on the splint surface. Even if parafunction continues the intervening splint will prevent damage to the teeth. It is important to motivate patients to wear their splints by stressing the long-term consequences of them not doing so.

Management of mandibular dysfunction
Many studies have shown that an occlusal splint may be beneficial in reducing the pain experienced in mandibular dysfunction.[8] Various theories have been put forward to explain the mechanism involved. One of the more common theories is that in lowering masticatory muscle activity, a splint will effectively reduce the build-up of metabolic waste products which may result in restricting muscle pain and spasm. While there is no doubt that many patients suffering from dysfunction who are treated with occlusal splints, do show a significant decrease in pain levels, it is far from clear that the therapeutic effect of the splint is responsible.[10] It is possible that a significant part of this improvement is achieved through the placebo effect (although there is some evidence that occlusal treatment with a splint does have a truly therapeutic effect[11,12]). Because of the difficulties dentists may experience in diagnosing the source of a patient's facial pain and the doubts which exist over the therapeutic effect of occlusal treatment, it is advisable to carry out only reversible occlusal treatment on such patients (splint therapy, not occlusal equilibration).

Pre-restorative stabilisation
The first part of this paper described the importance of occlusal stability and introduced the concept of reorganising the occlusion to create a new and stable ICP at the retruded position when stability is absent. When conforming to the existing ICP the maxillo-mandibular relationship to which restorations are made is easily and accurately determined by the intercuspation of the teeth. When reorganising it is necessary to locate and record the retruded position of the mandible and then mount both diagnostic and working casts on an articulator in this relationship. In the absence of stable ICP contacts this position is determined solely by the temporomandibular joints and associated neuromuscular system. It is essential that the patient's masticatory system is free from dysfunction, either internal derangement or extra-capsular muscle dysfunction, in order that a correct and reproducible retruded position can be recorded. A consistent position must be recorded before embarking upon restorative treatment. If not, it is likely that changes in the occlusal relationship may occur following tooth preparation and temporisation, or cementation of the new restorations. When reorganising the occlusion it is essential to precede restorative procedures with a period of splint therapy to ensure that a stable relationship has been achieved.

Creating space to restore worn anterior teeth
Figures 5 and 6 show a patient before and after splint therapy. At initial examination (fig. 5) the patient requested restoration of severely worn mandibular anterior teeth. It appeared that both ICP and the retruded position were coincident and that no space was available to correctly restore these teeth. After 1 month of wearing an occlusal splint (fig. 6), the mandible had repositioned posteriorly into a stable retruded position. This created space to enable the worn teeth to be properly restored. This repositioning occurred because the pre-existing discrepancy between RCP and ICP had been hidden by the patient's neuromuscular system.

Protection of new restorations from parafunction
The aetiology of parafunction is largely stress-related. It is likely that patients will continue to brux and clench after restoration of worn teeth. It is highly advisable for them to wear a post-restorative splint to protect their new restorations from damage. This should be made clear to the patient before treatment begins.

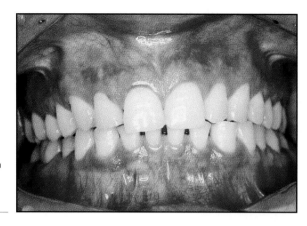

Fig. 5 The intercuspal position showing contact between worn mandibular incisal edges and the opposing teeth

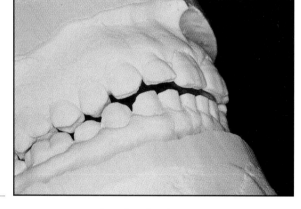

Fig. 6 One month of occlusal splint therapy resulting in posterior repositioning of the mandible

Types of occlusal splint — advantages and disadvantages

Many types of occlusal splint have been advocated. They may be full or partial occlusal coverage, maxillary or mandibular, repositioning or stabilising, and made from a variety of different materials.

Choice of materials

The material of choice is laboratory-processed acrylic resin. It is a reasonably hard material which may be easily adjusted and is durable enough to serve as a protective nightguard. Resilient vacuformed vinyl splints are of limited use. Although quick and economic to make they are soon destroyed by determined bruxers. Their resilient surface is not amenable to the production and maintenance of the stable occlusion necessary to achieve muscle relaxation.[13] The use of hard metal alloys such as

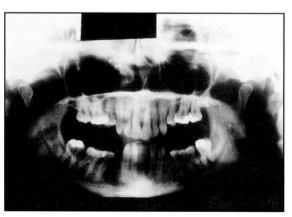

Fig. 7 The effect on tooth position of wearing a posterior onlay occlusal splint

cobalt/chrome to cover occlusal surfaces is highly inadvisable as it will result in increased wear of the opposing teeth.

Partial coverage splints

Occlusal splints must be worn continually, often for considerable periods of time to be effective. If a splint does not cover all the occlusal surfaces in an arch, unopposed teeth will continue to erupt creating an iatrogenic malocclusion. This applies to both anterior and posterior partial coverage splints and their use cannot therefore be recommended.

Figure 7 shows a radiograph of a patient who had worn a posterior onlay splint for about 1 year. When she closed into ICP, the posterior teeth were several millimetres apart (the thickness of the splint). The appliance provided no anterior coverage but had permitted the incisors and canines to supra-erupt, and led to intrusion of the posterior segments. An anterior splint would permit the posterior teeth to erupt, so that when the splint was removed the anterior teeth would be apart and anterior guidance would have been lost. In this series a technique will be described where a form of anterior splint (Dahl appliance) is used to gain space to restore worn anterior teeth. This is entirely different as it is a carefully planned procedure in which the anterior space created is filled and guidance restored with restorations placed on the severely worn teeth.

Maxillary or mandibular splints?

Providing the requirements of full occlusal coverage, posterior stability, anterior guidance and use of an appropriate material are met, it matters little whether a splint is made on the maxillary or mandibular arch. In Class I and II incisor relationships it is easier to produce an ideal occlusion on a maxillary appliance while the converse is true in Class III situations.

Stabilisation versus repositioning splints

Ramjford and Ash originally described the stabilisation or Michigan-type splint for which detailed fabrication and use will be covered in the final section of the paper. It is a full coverage maxillary splint made from laboratory processed acrylic resin which provides anterior disclusion and stable ICP contacts between a generally flat surface and the opposing teeth. It does not seek to actively reposition the mandible into a predetermined position. It is impossible at the outset to predict the extent and direction of mandibular repositioning, and any attempt to guide the mandible more actively with the splint may actually prevent stabilisation of the retruded position.

Stabilisation splints, through causing muscle relaxation, may also aid the repositioning of a displaced meniscus providing the displacement is neither too severe nor too longstanding.

The use of splints which seek to reposition the mandible in a predetermined position has been advocated, particularly in cases of internal derangement where some studies have shown them to be more effective than stabilisation splints.[14] They possess occlusal surfaces with well-defined fossae into which the opposing teeth locate with the mandible in the desired position. The problem with the use of such splints is that they may not achieve the desired masticatory muscle relaxation: also it is exceptionally difficult if not impossible to predict exactly the position in which the mandible should be located. This position is generally downward and forward from the habitual ICP, the rationale being that the stress on the disrupted joint components will be relieved, permitting them to gradually realign.[15] They also have the considerable disadvantage that following repositioning of the meniscus the patient may be left with a posterior open bite. If this occurs occlusal contacts may gradually re-establish through supra-eruption. Sometimes orthodontic treatment may be necessary to re-establish occlusal stability.

Because of the difficulties in use and the possible irreversible changes which may be caused to the patient's occlusion, the use of these appliances in general practice is recommended only with caution and in experienced hands.

Fabrication, fitting, adjusting and monitoring a Michigan splint

Fabrication

Maxillary and mandibular full arch alginate impressions are made in metal rimlock trays. The impressions should be quickly poured with the occlusal surfaces downward to ensure accurate reproduction of surface detail. While the stone is setting the poured impressions must be stored in a humid atmosphere. A Tupperware box containing moist paper towels is ideal. When the impressions are removed, the casts should be left to dry for 24 hours; if articulated too soon, the damp stone surfaces will be abraded and rendered inaccurate.

The casts should be mounted in a semi-adjustable articulator using a facebow record to mount the maxillary cast and an interocclusal record taken on the retruded axis to establish the maxillo-mandibular relation. The interocclusal registration is a pre-contact record using a rim of extra hard wax which fits accurately over the maxillary teeth without contacting the soft tissues. A fluid recording medium (Kerrs Tempbond) is applied to the lower surface to register the cusp tips of the mandibular teeth on closure. Control of the mandible is improved by means of a traditional anterior jig which prevents the teeth from coming into contact making manipulation of the mandible easier and determining the vertical dimension of the record.

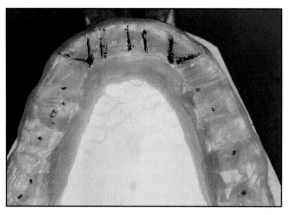

Fig. 8 Wax-up of occlusal splint on articulator showing contacts and anterior guidance

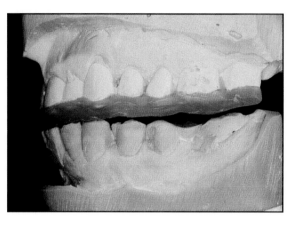

Fig. 9 Lateral view of splint wax-up showing disclusion of posterior teeth in lateral excursion

The incisal pin of the articulator is adjusted to provide a space of a roughly 2 mm between the most posterior teeth, and the outline of the splint drawn on the maxillary cast in pencil. It should extend about 3 mm onto the palatal soft tissues and wrap just over the buccal cusps and incisal edges. The splint will be retained by clipping into proximal, buccal and lingual undercuts and so these should not be blocked out prior to waxing. Two thicknesses of pink baseplate wax are softened and adapted over the cast and then trimmed to the pencil outline. The articulator is closed together until the incisal pin contacts the incisal table, establishing the vertical dimension of occlusion of the splint. The wax is then trimmed and the occlusion adjusted (articulating paper can be used on the wax) to establish the desired occlusion (fig. 8). Contacts are established between the flat surface of the splint and all opposing teeth while a shallow, smooth con-

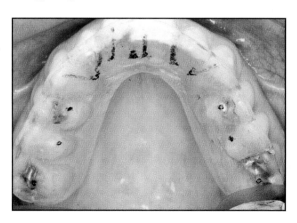

Fig. 10 Adjusted splint — holding contacts (Black), lateral canine guidance (Red), and protrusive (Green)

1 Schaerer P, Stallard R E, Zander H A, Occlusal interferences and mastication; an electromyographic study. *J Prosthet Dent* 1967; 17: 438-449.

2 Rankow K, Carlsson K, Edlund J, Oberg T. The effect of an occlusal interference on the masticatory system. *Odont Revy* 1976; 27: 245-256.

3 Howat A P, Capp N J, Barrett N V J. *A colour atlas of occlusion and malocclusion.* London: Wolfe Publishing Ltd, 1991. Chapters 2,4,10,11.

4 Furstman L. The effect of loss of occlusion upon the mandibular joint. *Am J Orthod* 1965; 51:1245.

5 Ramjford S P, Walden J M, Enlow R D. Unilateral function and the temporomandibular joint in Rhesus Monkeys. *Oral surg* 1971; 32: 237.

6 Solberg W K, Clark G T, Rugh J D. Nocturnal electromyographic evaluation of bruxism patients undergoing short-term splint therapy. *J Oral Rehab* 1975; 12: 215-223.

7 Beard C C, Clayton J A. Effects of occlusal splint therapy on TMJ dysfunctions. *J Prosthet Dent* 1980; 44: 324.

8 Shields J M, Clayton J A, Sindledecker L D. Using pantographic tracings to detect TM J and muscle dysfunctions. *J Prosthet Dent* 1978; 39: 80.

9 Crispin B J, Myers G E, Clayton J A. Effects of occlusal therapy on pantographic reproducibility of mandibular border movements. *J Prosthet Dent* 1978; 40: 29-34.

10 Feinmann C, Harris M. Psychogenic facial pain — Parts I & II. *Br Dent J* 1984; 156: 165, 205.

11 Forsell H, Kirveskari P, Kangasniemi P. Changes in headache after treatment of mandibular dysfunction Cephalagia. 1985; 5: 229-36.

12 Forsell H, Kirveskari P, Kangasniemi P. Response to occlusal treatment in headache patients previously treated by mock occlusal adjustment. *Acta Odont Scand* 1987; 45: 77-80.

13 Nevarro E, Barghi N, Rej R. Clinical evaluation of maxillary hard and resilient occlusal splints. *J Dent Res* Abstract 1246. Special Issue March 1985.

14 Anderson G, Schulte J, Goodkind R. Comparative study of two treatment methods for internal derangement of the temporomandibular joint. *J Prosthet Dent* 1985; 53: 392-397.

15 Solberg W. K. *Temporomandibular disorders.* London: BDJ Handbook, 1986, p96.

16 Capp N J. Temporomandibular joint dysfunction — its relevance to restorative dentistry. Part 2: splint therapy and restorative considerations. *Rest Dent* 1986; 2; 62-68.

cave ramp is built up in the anterior region to provide immediate, but smooth, disclusion of the posterior teeth on mandibular movement (fig. 9).

Once complete, the maxillary cast is removed from the articulator invested in a flask, the wax boiled out, and then the mould packed with clear acrylic resin which is then processed. The splint is devested, cleaned, trimmed and polished and is then ready for fitting.

Fitting and adjustment

To fit and adjust an occlusal splint will take about 30 minutes. Firstly, the retention is tested and if too tight, acrylic resin is removed with a laboratory carbide bur from the undercut areas around the teeth until the splint seats fully and is adequately retentive. Should the splint exhibit any rocking or lack of seating despite adjustment, it is likely that the casts were inaccurate and new impressions should be made.

Accurate occlusal adjustment requires the use of very thin articulating paper held taut in Millers forceps to ensure that only the actual areas of occlusal contact are marked. The adjustment of the splint is carried out using a large laboratory carbide bur which will adjust the contacts while maintaining a flat occlusal surface. The use of too small a bur will produce indentations in the splint which are undesirable.

Adjustment is carried out with the dental nurse holding two pieces of articulating paper in the patient's mouth and the dentist providing light guidance to the patient's chin with the patient being asked to 'rub forward and back' on the splint. This will guide the mandible toward the retruded position. After marking, the splint is removed and the contacts adjusted until all mandibular teeth make even contact on the splint surface with the mandible in the retruded position. It will probably be impossible at this stage to obtain the correct retruded position because of the state of the patient's neuromuscular system and TMJ's.

Following establishment of these contacts, the splint is adjusted in lateral and protrusive movements. In lateral movements, the guidance is provided by contact between the mandibular canines and the splint surface (fig. 10), which separates all the other teeth. In protrusive movements, disclusion is provided by even contact between the mandibular incisors and the splint (fig. 10). No other teeth should make contact outside ICP.

Once adjustment is complete, the patient is instructed in how to look after the splint and to wear it as much as possible.

Monitoring splint therapy

If an occlusal splint is being used only as a night guard to protect teeth or restorations it is advisable to review the patient after 7 days to check whether their occlusion has remained stable and to readjust if necessary. After this the splint should be checked at each routine examination.

If the splint is being used to treat mandibular dysfunction or for pre-restorative stabilisation the patient must be reviewed and the splint readjusted at weekly intervals for as long as is necessary to achieve a stable retruded position. The time necessary for this to occur may vary from a couple of weeks to several months.

At each adjustment the occlusion is re-examined and the splint readjusted to re-establish even contact and to eliminate excursive interferences. A stable relationship has been achieved when the occlusal contacts marked on the splint remain unchanged for two successive appointments.

If splint therapy were initiated to treat mandibular dysfunction no irreversible alteration to the patient's occlusion (equilibration) is generally needed. The patient may be gradually weaned off the splint but told to wear it if their discomfort returns which is often at times of stress.

If the aim of splint therapy was to stabilise the mandible prior to re-organised restorative treatment, stabilisation of the occlusion on the splint must be followed by an accurate mounting of diagnostic casts in the new maxillomandibular relationship. Monitoring the progress of splint therapy is usually carried out by observation of the occlusal contacts on the splint at each adjustment appointment. Prior to more complex restorative procedures and for the purposes of research, the effect the splint has on the stability of the retruded position and other mandibular border movements may be followed very precisely using pantographic tracings of mandibular border movements.[3,8,9]

The casts, once re-mounted, can then be used to plan and rehearse the restorative procedures. This may necessitate adjustment but will certainly involve diagnostic waxing.

Conclusions

Patients affected by tooth surface loss need protective management. This is based on the elimination, where possible, of the primary cause with careful selection and use of restorative materials to improve or preserve occlusal stability. Where loads on teeth are high, an occlusal splint can be a very effective way of limiting further wear. If preventive strategies have either not been introduced or not complied with, the dentition may be very worn and fixed restorations impossible to provide. Consequently, removable prostheses are frequently used to restore those severely affected by tooth surface loss, Part 4 of the series discusses the principles of their use.

The author is most grateful to Mosby-Year Book Europe Ltd for permission to use the illustrations in Figures 1, 2, 8 and 9.
This article is based on a presentation at The Medical Society of London on 2 November 1994 as part of the Alpha Omega lecture programme.

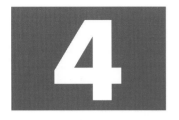

Removable prostheses

M. Faigenblum[1]

The previous article discussed changes in the occlusion that take place when teeth wear. Severe wear, particularly when coupled with tooth loss, can produce marked changes in the occlusal relationships and significant aesthetic deficit. A removable prosthesis may be the appropriate restorative approach particularly when wear is advanced. Determination of the correct vertical dimension for the occlusion and an appropriate jaw relationship form the basis of treatment whether this employs fixed or removable prostheses. Later articles will examine both adhesive and more traditional fixed approaches to restoration. However, this paper describes the use of removable appliances for restoring dentitions affected by tooth surface loss and how the aesthetic and technical difficulties created by the lack of space may be overcome.

The maintenance of anterior facial height by compensatory growth

The craniofacial complex is not a static entity in the adult;[1] there is evidence that growth, though slower than takes place during adolescence, continues into late middle age.[2] An aspect of such growth ie the increase in anterior facial height has been reported.[2–4] One of the mechanisms for this increase (in the absence of excessive tooth wear) is thought to be from the eruption of teeth because of an increase in alveolar height.[5,6]

Tallgren noted that with the complete dentition, anterior facial height tends to increase with age and that this increase is paralleled by the rest of the face height;[3] in other words, the free-way space (FWS) remains constant. This relationship appears to hold as long as there is no appreciable destructive change in the dentition.

Where uniform wear of the occlusal surfaces and incisal edges does take place, Sicher suggests that this is compensated by continuous vertical eruption and thus attrition does not affect the proportions of the face.[7] Niswonger (cited by Tallgren[3]) among others[6,8] supported this view. He found that 80% of severe wear cases had a normal FWS ie 3 mm.

However, there is a contrary view (Thompson,[4] Mershon,[9] and Kazis,[10]) which affirms that the FWS is affected by wear and its magnitude is proportional to the degree of attrition. Stern and Brayer[11] state that: 'Pathological changes of the occlusion may

occur when posterior tooth support is reduced or lost. In these cases, the mandible requires a new support which is usually found in the anterior region of the mouth. Consequently, an excessive occlusal load affects the anterior teeth. Such an event is known as 'occlusal collapse.' Russell,[12] supports this concept. He considers that an FWS in excess of 5–6 mm is abnormal and that the occlusal wear which has produced it, has occurred at a rate faster than the physiological mechanisms designed to compensate for it'. This presumption is disputed in a recent paper by Smith and Robb.[13]

These apparently contrasting opinions are reflected in the following clinical observations. Dawson is adamant that as wear does not decrease the occlusal vertical dimension (OVD), there is no case for its increase during treatment.[14] Nonetheless, he subsequently states that: 'If the contacting surface enamel is worn severely on both the upper and lower anterior teeth, there is sometimes no room to restore the surfaces... without either invading the pulp or increasing the vertical dimension. This type of problem is usually treated by opening the vertical'. Watson and Tulloch too, find a seeming paradox in relation to OVD. They comment, that: 'Clinically one frequently finds that despite considerable TSL there is very little interocclusal clearance...on the other hand...the extent of the freeway space is sometimes commensurate with a natural FWS together with the TSL'.

This apparent conflict can be resolved by modifying Pindborg's original classification of TSL.[16] The latter makes a distinction between generalised and localised tooth wear.[12,16]

- *Compensated TSL:* Tooth surface loss without loss of OVD. It generally involves a complete or nearly complete dentition and the free-way space remains within the normal range.
- *Non-compensated TSL:* Tooth surface loss leading to the loss of OVD. This is often confined to the anterior segments and associated with a lack of posterior occlusion. The rate of wear, confined to a smaller number of teeth, results in an apparent lack of compensatory eruption and the free-way space is greater than normal.

With compensated TSL, the occlusal plane is generally not in doubt. During treatment, the increase in vertical dimension is usually

Reconstruction of the dentition extensively damaged through tooth surface loss may require the use of removable prostheses. This can be the most appropriate type of treatment when either the teeth are very severely worn or the patient wishes a simpler and more economical approach than a fixed reconstruction.

[1]*Honorary Clinical Senior Lecturer, Department of Prosthetic Dentistry, Eastman Dental Institute for Oral Healthcare Sciences, University of London, 256 Gray's Inn Road, London WC1X 8LD and Specialist in Prosthodontics, 25 Devonshire Place, London W1N 1PD*

dependent on the space required to restore the teeth. Repositioning of the mandible will re-establish a normal FWS but the anterior lower facial height (ALFH) will be increased.

With non-compensated TSL, the collapse of ALFH necessitates an increase in the vertical dimension to restore the subjects to their presumed, original OVD before TSL took place.

As patients with compensated TSL rarely present for removable partial denture (RPD) treatment, the following discussion will, in the main, be directed to non-compensated TSL.

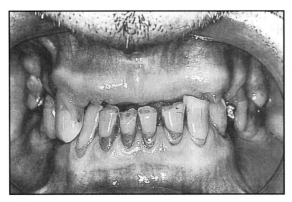

Fig. 1 Anterior view of a patient's intercuspal position (ICP) showing exceptionally heavy wear of the upper incisors. Note the shiny surface of the apparently non-functional amalgam surface on the |5

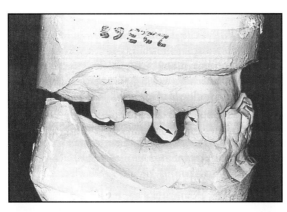

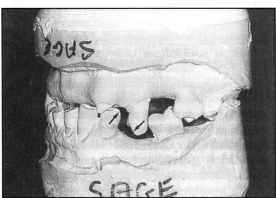

Fig. 2a and 2b Lateral views of the casts in ICP. The posterior segments are 'collapsed' and there appears to be gross over-eruption. Note the relationship of the apparently over-erupted upper second premolar teeth to the lower first premolar. The arrows indicate the presence of wear facets

Assessment of non-compensated TSL

The patient affected by non-compensated TSL with loss of facial height poses the same problem as in complete denture prosthodontics; how to establish a functional OVD. The absence of an acceptable occlusal plane also complicates the determination of an appropriate intercuspal position (ICP).

Two characteristics may be of value in guiding the operator toward the optimal retruded axis position (RAP) and hence a convenient occlusal vertical dimension (OVD).[17]

Firstly, when teeth are found distal to the worn anterior surfaces, a facet may be present which often appears to be coincident with the retruded contact position (RCP). (It will be obvious if this first contact is a result of over-eruption.) Secondly, this contact will frequently produce an acceptable OVD. This can be confirmed by reference to the patient's appearance and in particular to an unstrained relationship of the lips in apposition.

Figures 1 to 5 illustrate this suggestion. The unstable contacts seen in figures 3a and b may be responsible for deflecting the mandible forward into ICP, a position to which the functional movements of mastication and swallowing are normally directed.[18] The posterior contacts no longer being used, the anterior teeth suffer progressive wear which is probably a combination of attrition and erosion.[19] When the mandible is held at the retruded contact position, the original occlusal plane, common to both arches, can be envisaged and there is no longer any evidence of significant over-eruption. The outline of anterior tooth form can be extrapolated from the proportions of the remaining tooth structure and the available interarch space (fig. 4); a diagnostic wax-up will show this more accurately.

Thus, an examination of the casts mounted in RCP, will often allow the operator to visualise the degree of tooth loss and the extent of restoration required. This can be the starting point for the proposed restoration.

Treatment of non-compensated TSL

The following is a schematic outline for the treatment of TSL with a removable prostheses. Management can be divided into three stages:
1. Preliminary investigations
2. Restorative phase
3. Maintenance.

Preliminary investigations:
1. Routine examination
2. Note the presence and position of facets and their relationship on opposing teeth (this is most easily seen on the casts)
3. Assess the amount of free-way space (FWS)
4. Manipulate the mandible into RCP and observe the effect on the facial appearance
5. Make impressions of the complete arches

and verify the accuracy the resultant casts[20]

6. Make duplicates of these casts after blocking out undercuts

7. Using a measuring device (eg Willis Bite Gauge) record the rest vertical dimension (RVD)

8. Take an interocclusal record at a jaw separation approximating the RVD recorded

9. Note the occlusal vertical height (OVD) when the teeth are in ICP

10. Deduct the OVD from the RVD to obtain the FWS

11. With the casts mounted and the interocclusal record *in situ*, note the reading on the scale of the incisal pin (ie this is equivalent to the RVD, see 8 above)

12. Close the articulator until first tooth contact and again take note of the reading on the incisal pin. (If there is no posterior contact close the articulator until the upper and lower occlusal planes appear to coincide)

13. Close the articulator into ICP and note the reading at the incisal pin

14. Compare these results with those found *in vivo*. If the first contact (or coincidence of the occlusal plane) produces an acceptable FWS and facial appearance, use this as a guide for restoration

15. An occlusal splint is constructed, as described in Part 3 of this series. It is usually most convenient to construct a maxillary appliance. Little, if any, alterations should be made to the teeth at this stage. This is to allow abandonment of treatment with a minimum of recrimination. Teeth can be added to the splint, making it, in effect, an overlay denture. When adjustments and habituation have produced a satisfactory functional and aesthetic result, the next stage can be embarked upon.

2. Restorative phase

The OVD and ICP having been established by the upper occlusal splint, it is possible to envisage two situations:

1. Where the lower dentition produces a satisfactory occlusal plane, there is no need for a lower denture to complement the upper splint/denture unless there are specific reasons eg aesthetics

2. Where the loss of teeth and tooth substance in the lower arch have created a need for a lower denture to establish a harmonious occlusal plane. The occlusal splint having followed the irregular lower occlusal plane, it itself is unaesthetic as it overlays the teeth. Two methods can be used:

• The casts are articulated as described above and the lower denture is waxed up to meet the upper contacts, care being taken to present an harmonious occlusal plane to which the definitive upper denture can eventually

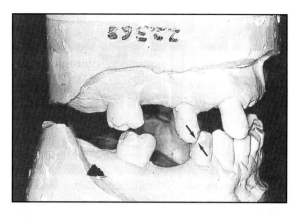

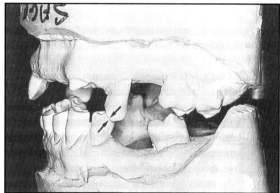

Fig. 3a and 3b Lateral views of the casts after the mandible has been guided into RCP. Note that the facets are now in contact and the apparent overeruption of the 7531578 has resolved into an acceptable occlusal plane

be made to occlude

• The lower cast is articulated against a cast of the occlusal splint. An idealised occlusal plane is set up, stone from the opposing cast being removed to allow this. The definitive lower denture is fitted and appropriate adjustments are made to the splint.

Choice of the denture base material

This will depend on various factors including the opposing materials and whether coverage is mainly on hard or soft tissue:

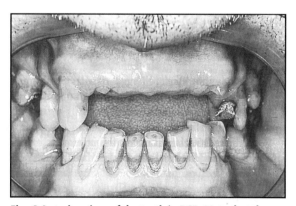

Fig. 4 Anterior view of the teeth in RCP. Note that the facet on the upper left premolar is on the amalgam restoration and its lustre indicates wear during function (figures 1 and 5). This is belied by its situation in ICP, as seen in figure 2b

1   Crothers A, Sandham A. Vertical height differences in subjects with severe dental wear. *Eur J Orthod* 1993; **15**: 519-525.

2   Behrent R G. *Growth in the aging craniofacial skeleton.* Craniofacial Growth series. Monograph No.17 Center for Human Growth and Development. Michigan: University of Michigan, Ann Arbor, 1985.

3   Tallgren A. Changes in adult face height due to ageing, wear and loss of teeth and prosthetic treatment. *Acta Odont Scand* 1957; **15**: Suppl.24, 73.

4   Thompson J L, Kendrick G S. Changes in the vertical dimension of the human male skull during the third and fourth decades of life. *Anat Rec* 1964; **27**: 209.

5   Manson J D. Passive eruption. *Dent Pract* 1963; **14**: 2-8.

6   Murphy T. Compensatory mechanisms in facial height adjustment to functional tooth attrition. *Aust Dent J* 1959; **4**: 312-323.

7   Sicher H. *Oral biology.* St Louis, CV Mosby Co. 1949 (in Tallgren 1957.)

8   Berry D C, Poole D F G. Attrition: possible mechanisms of compensation. *J Oral Rehabil* 1976; **3**: 201-206.

9   Mershon J V. Possibilities and limitations in the treatment of closed-bites. *Int J Orthodont* 1937; **23**: 581-589 (in Tallgren A. 1957).

10 Kazis H. Complete mouth rehabilitation through restoration of lost vertical dimension. *J Am Dent Ass* 1948; **37**: 19-39 (in Tallgren A. 1957).

11 Stern N, Brayer L. Collapse of the occlusion — aetiology, symptomatology and treatment. *J Oral Rehabil* 1975; **2**: 1-19.

12 Russell M D. The distinction between physiological and pathological attrition: a review. *Ir Dent Assoc* 1987; **33**: 23.

13 Smith B G N, Robb N D. The prevalence of toothwear in 1007 dental patients. *J Oral Rehabil* 1996; **23**: 232-239.

14 Dawson P. *Evaluation, diagnosis and treatment of occlusal problems.* 2nd ed. Mosby-Toronto, 1989.

15 Watson I B, Tulloch E N. Clinical assessment of cases of tooth surface loss. *Br Dent J* 1985; **159**:144-148.

16 Pindborg J J. *Pathology of dental hard tissues.* pp300-309. Copenhagen: Munksgaard, 1970.

17 Hemmings K W, Howlett J A, Woodley N J, *et al.* Partial dentures for patients with advanced tooth wear. *Dent Update* 1995; **22**: 52-59.

18 Ramfjord S P. Bruxism, a clinical and electromyographic study. *JADA* 1961; **62**: 21-44.

19 Lewis K J, Smith B G N. The relationship of erosion and attrition in extensive tooth tissue loss. *Br Dent J* 1973; **135**: 400-404.

20 Faigenblum M J. Advice on producing an accurate impression and working cast for construction of partial dentures. *Br Dent J* 1985; **159**: 45-46.

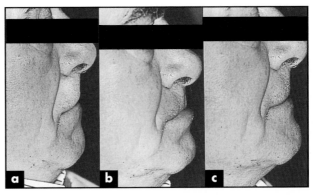

Fig. 5 The patient's profile is seen in his rest position (fig. 5b) and at the RCP (fig. 5c). In ICP the patient's lower anterior facial height is very much reduced. However, at RCP the face takes on a more normal appearance. In particular note that the lips appear to be in unstrained contact

- Because a well-supported denture is of primary importance; the best design for the definitive lower denture is based on a metal framework
- The definitive upper denture will benefit from a metal construction if the splint has shown signs of excessive wear resulting in breakage
- The final prosthesis can be veneered over its entire occlusal surface with cobalt chromium which will strengthen the appliance and avoid the need to attempt the reproduction of the appearance and functional occlusion *de novo*. When using cobalt chromium attention must be paid to the likelihood that the opposing arch may suffer accelerated wear.

Management of the appearance
Two options are available for restoring the worn teeth:

1. Complete facings with or without a flange
2. Butt joint.

The materials can be purpose-made acrylic facings, hollowed-out denture teeth or custom made in the mouth with autopolymerising resin, composite, or light curing resin. An opaquer may be necessary to mask the colour of a metal base. In the latter case, special provisions will also need to be made for retention either mechanically or chemically.

The choice of restoration will depend upon:
- Path of insertion of the denture
- The ability of the lip to tolerate labial coverage of the teeth
- The height of the lip during function ie if the butt joint is visible
- The occlusion
- The ability to match the colour of the overlaid tooth with the restorative material.

Maintenance
One objective of treatment is to produce an appliance which is resistant to degradation but nonetheless is capable of simple servicing at routine checkups. Overlay dentures will normally be worn at night to prevent parafunctional attrition of the teeth. If it is thought that this will place the denture at too much risk an occlusal splint may be substituted.

Conclusion
The article has discussed the effects of tooth surface loss on anterior facial height and how this can be related to the distribution of wear within the mouth. Identification of the changes that have taken place is important in making a complete assessment of the patient and forming a restorative plan. Removable appliances may be the treatment of choice for some individuals, particularly when the time and cost of fixed restorations are considered. The complexities of treatment of the severely worn dentition serve to re-emphasise the importance of effective prevention as discussed in the first three parts of this series. There may also be a case for early restoration to prevent the extensive damage to the teeth which necessitates extensive reconstruction. Parts 1 and 2 mentioned a possible role for early restorative intervention to minimise further wear: this is sometimes considered controversial as concerns have been expressed over wear continuing around the margins of restorations. However, there is merit in such an approach, particularly if the restorative techniques are relatively non-invasive and it is coupled with an overall preventive approach. Part 5 examines the role of adhesive dentistry in the management of the worn dentition.

This article is based on a presentation at The Medical Society of London on 15 December 1994 as part of the Alpha Omega lecture programme.

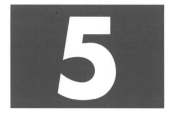

Adhesive techniques

P. A. King[1]

This paper describes the use of adhesive techniques to restore teeth previously affected by tooth surface loss so avoiding the need to remove sound tooth tissue.

A number of the previous articles have described the importance of early diagnosis of tooth surface loss and not allowing wear to become too advanced before some form of restoration is provided. The early use of traditional restorations (such as crowns) is very correctly frowned upon if the cause of the wear is either not known or reasonably well-controlled as their prognosis in the presence of continuing wear is poor. The development of adhesive dentistry has simplified much of the restorative care of people with worn teeth. It has substituted for many of the traditional treatment strategies. The conservative nature of adhesive procedures and their relative reversibility make them attractive both for restoring worn teeth and protecting them from further wear.

Treatment is sometimes provided at an early stage: this can be indicated when the cause of the wear resists diagnosis, tooth surface loss is ongoing despite a preventive regime or the patient's symptoms have not responded to initial management. This article outlines the broad range of dental materials and adhesive techniques currently available for restoring worn teeth. The emphasis is placed on the application of techniques rather than any specific restorative material as the latter change constantly as new developments are made.

The introduction to the dental profession of the acid-etch technique using phosphoric acid in the early 1960s, began the modern development of adhesive materials and techniques. The later introduction of dentine bonding agents, silane primers, and composite resin luting cements has made possible predictable adhesion between dental and tissues and a variety of materials such as composite resins, ceramics and metal alloys.

Worn teeth are not particularly difficult to restore when the materials are used in non-occluding areas. Where a functional surface has become worn and requires restoration, the main problem is one of a lack of space for the restorative material without preparing an already worn tooth. The traditional prosthodontic approach has often been to restore all the teeth in one or both arches to increase the occlusal vertical dimension. This can require the unnecessary treatment of teeth which have not been greatly affected by wear but require restoration to bring them into contact with antagonists at the new vertical dimension of occlusion.

One of the most significant advances in treatment has been the ability to re-create the space lost by the teeth as they wear. It is based on the use of a bite-plane appliance localised to the worn teeth. This intrudes them and their antagonists while encouraging the eruption of those taken out of contact by the appliance. Used in combination with adhesive restorative techniques this method has provided an extremely conservative approach to the restorative management of worn teeth.

The article describes the use of appliances to create the space necessary for restoration and the immediate provision of the final restorations which are fitted leaving the occlusion intentionally 'high'; and allowing axial tooth movement to re-establish complete occlusion.

Restorative management of tooth surface loss

Cervical tooth wear

These lesions present in a variety of forms depending on the type and severity of the causative factors. Not all lesions require restoration, but if aesthetics, sensitivity, or structural considerations dictate then some form of adhesive restoration will usually be most suitable.

There is a plethora of tooth-coloured restorative materials now available. Materials can either be composite resin or glass-ionomer based, or a combination of both; either in a layered technique with the individual materials or as a resin-modified glass ionomer cement. The choice of materials can be bewildering, with new materials and techniques seemingly introduced to the market on a weekly basis.[1]

There are a number of approaches to bonding restorations to cervical tooth tissue.[2] For lesions with margins that are still confined to enamel the use of a microfine or polishable composite resin, in conjunction with acid etched enamel, will produce aesthetic and durable results. Unfortunately, most cervical lesion margins are not confined to enamel and usually involve root cementum and dentine. In this situation dentine bonding is required, usually in the form of a bonding agent in combination with a composite resin or a glass ionomer cement.

In situations where aesthetics are paramount then a polishable composite resin

[1]Consultant in Restorative Dentistry, University of Bristol Dental Hospital, Lower Maudlin Street, Bristol BS1 2LY

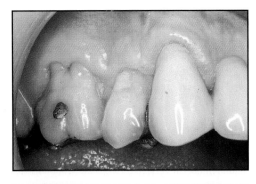

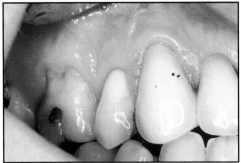

Fig. 1a,b Cervical tooth wear lesion affecting the upper right first premolar tooth restored with a light-activated resin-modified glass ionomer cement

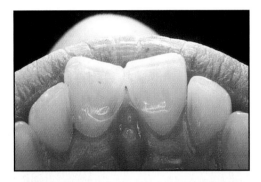

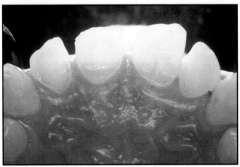

Fig. 2a,b Typical examples of localised anterior tooth wear predominantly due to acid erosion

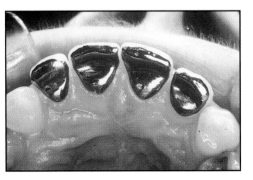

Fig. 3 Maxillary incisor teeth restored with resin-bonded nickel chromium-alloy palatal veneers

remains the material of choice. However, despite ongoing improvements there is still a question over the longer term durability of the resin-dentine bond.

Where lesions are not highly visible (perhaps involving root surface), a glass ionomer material may prove to be more appropriate. The dynamic bond of glass ionomer cements to both dentine and enamel through an ionic exchange provides the opportunity for continual repair of the adhesive bond at the tooth and cement interface. There is also the additional benefit of fluoride ion release from the glass ionomer cement reducing the possibility of marginal caries in susceptible individuals.

Although much improved in recent years, the colour properties of conventional glass ionomer cements are not ideal. In deeper cervical lesions however it is possible to consider a layered technique combining the adhesive properties of the glass ionomer cement with the superior colour properties of a polishable composite resin. The new generation of light-activated resin-modified glass ionomer materials combine some of the better properties of composite resin and conventional glass ionomer cements. The command set, improved colour and easier finishing of some of these newer materials allow the opportunity to provide very acceptable conservative restorations for cervical tooth wear lesions (fig. 1). Only longer term observation and assessment will determine how durable these newer materials will prove.

Anterior tooth wear

Localised tooth wear may affect just the anterior teeth. This is often seen in younger age groups where it is primarily caused by acid erosion, characteristically affecting the palatal aspects of the upper anterior teeth (fig. 2).

If only the palatal surfaces need restoring, the use of adhesive metal veneers is an acceptable method.[3,4] Nickel-chromium alloys (fig. 3) as used in resin-bonded bridge frameworks, or heat treated gold alloys (fig. 4) are appropriate. The decision between the two materials is based on the improved bond strength of resin to the nickel/chromium alloy versus the easier working properties and wear characteristics of the gold alloy.

Tooth preparation is minimal, usually restricted to smoothing the incisal and palatal peripheral enamel margins. Where there has been relatively deep erosion of the palatal surface it is often advisable to block out the deeper aspects of the cavity with either a glass ionomer cement alone or with a calcium hydroxide liner beneath it. This may offer some protection to the pulpal tissues and helps the laboratory and cementation procedures. Laboratory fabrication of the metal alloy veneers is either directly on a refractory working cast or using a wax/resin 'lift-off' technique.

When restoring worn anterior teeth, creation of the interocclusal space is usually required to accommodate the restorative material. As the tooth structure is already compromised avoiding further tooth reduction to create space is highly desirable. Orthodontic tooth movement using a Dahl anterior appliance is a well established method of achieving interocclusal space.[5] This is a predictable method although there are some disadvantages, not least the increased treatment time and extra laboratory procedures.

An alternative approach, based on similar principles to the Dahl appliance, is to deliberately design and construct the palatal veneers in such a manner that they are cemented initially 'high' in occlusion. Predictable tooth movement is enhanced if a positive cingulum contact can be achieved with the occluding lower incisor teeth in an attempt to direct forces along the long axes of the contacting teeth.

Luting agents can either be resin-based or a glass ionomer cement. The author's preference in most circumstances is for resin capable of adhesion to both tooth structure and metal oxide. By using opaque variants, greying of the incisal third caused by the underlying palatal metal veneer may be avoided. Rubber dam isolation is used wherever possible. Prior to cementation the fitting surface of the metal alloy is prepared using 50 micrometre aluminium oxide air abrasion. An acceptable adhesive bond using gold alloy veneers is achieved if the surface is additionally heat treated.[6]

Location of the veneers during cementation can be made easier by extending the metal coverage onto the incisal edges. This design is also likely to reduce the opportunity of debonding during function by offering some increased resistance to shearing loads and by covering a greater surface area of available tooth structure. Any potentially unaesthetic display of incisal metal can often be disguised by dulling the polished metal using an intra-oral air abrasive.

A step-by-step description of this particular clinical technique is shown in Table 1.

Although the use of metal palatal veneers is an excellent conservative method of managing localised anterior tooth wear, it is not possible to improve the appearance of lost incisal and labial tooth tissue. In these circumstances the initial build-up of the incisal portion with a composite resin, followed by the metal veneer to cover both tooth tissue and composite resin is a relatively straightforward variation on the technique.[7,8] One of the major disadvantages is that the composite resin will deteriorate and eventually require repair or replacement. An alternative approach is to restore the labial portion of the worn tooth with a porcelain laminate veneer in conjunction with a metal alloy veneer palatally.[9] However, careful consideration should be given to the provision of a more

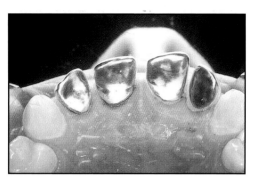

Fig. 4 Maxillary incisor teeth as shown in figure 2b restored with resin-bonded gold alloy palatal veneers

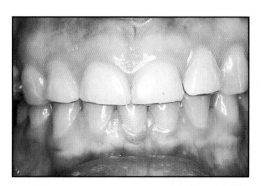

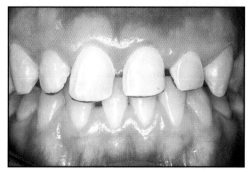

Fig. 5a,b Anterior appearance of resin-bonded gold alloy palatal veneers as shown in figures 3 and 4

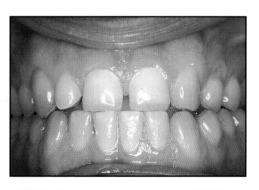

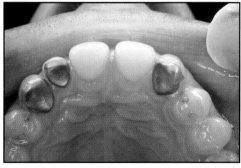

Fig. 6a,b The appearance of resin-bonded porcelain veneers used to restore the worn incisal and palatal surfaces of the maxillary central incisor teeth (resin-bonded gold alloy veneers were used on the remaining worn anterior teeth)

Table 1 Stepwise approach to the construction of resin-bonded metal alloy palatal veneers

- Minimal tooth preparation — smooth peripheral enamel margins including the incisal edges
- Line out any deep erosive/abrasive lesions
- Full arch elastomeric working impression, opposing arch alginate impression, and inter-occlusal record and facebow transfer as appropriate
- Laboratory construction of palatal metal alloy veneers either directly on a refractory cast or using a die-stone cast with a wax/resin 'lift-off' technique, prior to investing and casting in either type III gold alloy or nickel-chrome alloy
- Try in of metal alloy veneers ensuring good marginal fit, carrying out any minor adjustments as necessary
- Prepare metal alloy fitting surface with 50 micron aluminium oxide/air abrasive (laboratory or chairside), followed ideally by heat treatment in an air fired furnace at 400°C for 4 minutes (if using type III gold alloy laboratory)
- Rubber dam isolation of teeth (modified if necessary), and clean surface with pumice and water
- Acid treatment of enamel and dentine, thoroughly rinsed with water and dried, followed by the application of a dentine primer if significant area of dentine involved
- Application of composite resin luting agent, mixed according to manufacturer's instructions, applied to the veneer, followed by careful seating and removal of excess cement
- Refine occlusal contact on the veneer restorations
- Finish veneer margins with a combination of multi-fluted tungsten carbide burs and polishing wheels under full water spray
- Continue to monitor and refine occlusal contacts on veneer restorations

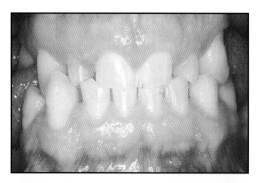

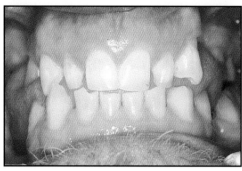

Fig. 7a,b Advanced anterior tooth wear combined with an unfavourable occlusal relationship restored as an interim measure with a direct acid-etch retained composite resin

conventional full coverage crown or possibly a resin-bonded minimal crown restoration.[10]

Some authors[11,12] recommend the use of porcelain laminate veneer restorations to restore both the incisal and palatal worn tooth tissue (fig. 6). There are however difficulties with this technique in that greater inter-occlusal space is required to accommodate the porcelain material, and it is often very difficult to disguise the junction between the incisal porcelain and remaining tooth structure on the labial aspect of the tooth. A similar, and very conservative alternative is to restore the incisal and palatal surfaces with direct acid-etch retained composite resin. This technique can be very useful as an interim measure and allows for the possibility of more involved and complex procedures in the form of conventional crowns to be considered at a later date (fig. 7).

In situations where the anterior tooth wear is mainly because of attrition, and the palatal surface is relatively unaffected, it may be possible to restore the incisal and labial surfaces with a partial porcelain laminate veneer. However, a sufficient space to allow restoration is necessary. This could be achieved locally using a Dahl appliance or if the posterior occlusion requires restoration by increasing the vertical dimension of occlusion.

Posterior tooth wear

Tooth wear affecting only posterior teeth is usually part of a generalised condition affecting the whole dentition. Occasionally the pattern of this tooth wear is such that individual posterior teeth may require restoration. If aesthetics are not paramount, a resin-bonded heat-treated gold alloy restoration can be advantageous.[13] These are useful where retention and resistance form for conventional crowns are particularly

compromised, and there is a desire to avoid adjunctive treatment such as periodontal crown lengthening.

Tooth preparation should be minimal. To help with the location of the onlay restoration there is some value in preparing an indentation on the occlusal surface of the tooth prior to the working impression. Ideally existing amalgam restorations should be replaced with either composite resin or glass ionomer cement to enhance the overall bond strength. Difficulties arise however with large proximal cavities which finish cervically on the root cementum. It may be difficult to maintain the adhesive bond in this area and a conventional cast restoration becomes more appropriate.

In generalised tooth wear where there are indications to consider a full mouth reconstruction of the dentition, the use of adhesive onlay restorations can be of value.[14] Space to restore worn anterior teeth either by adhesive or conventional methods can be obtained by an overall increase in occlusal vertical dimension. This allows the opportunity to restore the posterior teeth to re-establish occlusal stability. Restoring posterior quadrants with adhesive onlays is a conservative method, although it is not always possible to create sufficient inter-occlusal space by increasing the vertical dimension alone, particularly if opposing occluding surfaces in the molar regions need to be restored. In these circumstances some occlusal tooth reduction may also be necessary. Where space is at a premium the selection of a gold alloy as opposed to

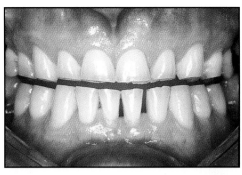

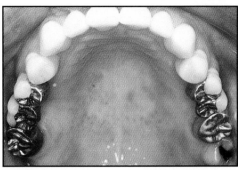

porcelain will be advantageous. Because of the normal arc of mandibular closure there will often be more space available in the premolar regions allowing the opportunity to use more aesthetic restorations (fig. 9). Aesthetic demand is often greater for occlusal surfaces in the mandibular arch.

In selected cases it is possible to consider a full mouth reconstruction of the worn dentition using resin-bonded ceramic restorations (fig. 10). The longer term durability, particularly of the posterior onlay restorations remains unpredictable and characteristically small fracture lines can appear in time which may eventually result in catastrophic failure.

New techniques bring with them new difficulties and challenges. The use of adhesive onlay restorations in managing the worn dentition is no exception. Temporisation following tooth preparation can be problematic. Procedures involving complete resin bonding of the temporary restoration to the underlying tooth tissue may compromise the subsequent adhesive bond for the final restoration. There is also a risk of damage to the tooth preparation during the removal of the interim restoration. Conversely using a less adhesive material or technique may result in the early loss of any temporary restorations with the possible consequences of unplanned tooth movement. Laboratory manufactured acrylic or composite resin quadrant splinted temporary restorations cemented with a composite resin lute to spot etched enamel have proved to be a reasonably reliable but expensive technique.

Checking the occlusal relationship at the try-in stage can also be difficult because of the relative lack of retention of the restorations before cementation. It is therefore critical that accurate jaw records are secured to allow precise mounting of the casts in an articulator. Attention to detail at this stage will usually reduce the need for any major adjustment to the restorations following cementation.

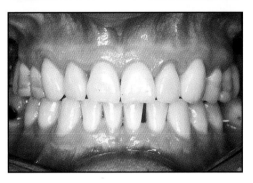

Fig. 8a–c 55-year-old male with moderate tooth wear (primarily tooth /tooth attrition in nature) who was concerned with the appearance of the upper anterior teeth. The maxillary arch was restored at an increase in occlusal vertical dimension with porcelain laminate veneers in the anterior segment, resin-bonded porcelain onlays for the first premolar teeth, and resin-bonded bridgework in the posterior segments. A conventional gold alloy casting was constructed for the extensively restored left first molar tooth

1   Willems G, Lambrechts P, Braem M, Vanherle G. Composite resins in the 21st century. *Quintessence Int* 1993; **24**: 641-658.

2   Watson T F, Bartlett D W. Adhesive systems: composites, dentine bonding agents and glass ionomers. *Br Dent J* 1994; **176**: 227-231.

3   Hussey D L, Irwin C R, Kime D L. Treatment of anterior tooth wear with gold palatal veneers. *Br Dent J* 1994; **176**: 422-425.

4   Darbar U R. Treatment of palatal erosive wear by using oxidised gold veneers: a case report. *Quintessence Int* 1994; **25**: 195-197.

5   Dahl B L, Krogstad O, Karlsen K. An alternative treatment in cases with advanced attrition. *J Oral Rehabil* 1975; **2**: 209-214.

6   Tanaka T, Atsuta M, Nakabayashi N, Masuhara E. Surface treatment of gold alloys for adhesion. *J Prosthet Dent* 1988; **60**: 271-279.

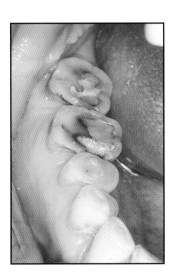

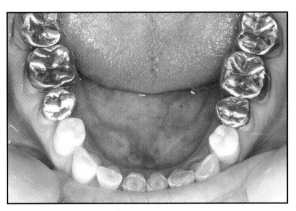

Fig. 9 a,b Worn mandibular posterior teeth restored with resin-bonded gold alloy and indirect composite resin onlays at an increase in occlusal vertical dimension

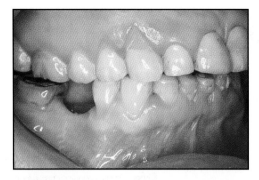

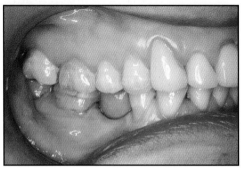

Fig. 10a,b 63-year-old female with moderate/advanced tooth wear of mixed aetiology. The maxillary and mandibular teeth were restored at an overall increase in occlusal vertical dimension with resin-bonded porcelain laminate veneers in the anterior region and resin-bonded cast ceramic onlays in the posterior segments

As ceramic technology improves and stronger, less abrasive, castable materials become available it may be more realistic to consider resin-bonded ceramic restorations when managing patients with generalised tooth wear.

Conclusions

A broad range of adhesive restorative options has been described. Many of these have used composite resin or other tooth-coloured filling materials which are likely to have a shorter life-span than those made of cast metal or metal-ceramic. However, the virtual absence of tooth preparation can make such restorations a very attractive option. Unfortunately, such a conservative approach is not always possible and there remain frequent indications for using conventional crowns to restore worn teeth. These traditional and sometimes more complex procedures will be described toward the end of the series. Where such treatment is contemplated, reasonable outcomes must be based on sound prevention and maintenance. In the next two articles, the characteristics of effective preventive regimes are first described while appropriately this is followed by a paper devoted to the causes and management of failures in crown and bridgework.

This article is based on a presentation at The Medical Society of London on 18 January 1995 as part of the Alpha Omega lecture programme.

7 Foreman P C. Resin-bonded acid-etched onlays in two cases of gross attrition. *Dent Update* 1988; **15**: 150-153.

8 Creugers H C, Kayser A F. The use of adhesive metal partial crowns to restore attrition defects: a case report. *Quintessence Int* 1992; **23**: 245-248.

9 Cheung S P, Dimmer A. Management of the worn dentition: a further use for the resin-bonded cast metal restoration. *Restor Dent* 1988; **4**: 76-78.

10 Holmes R, Dan Sneed W. Treatment of severe chemomechanical erosion using castable ceramic restorations and a new dentin/enamel bonding system: a case report. *Quintessence Int* 1990; **21**: 863-867.

11 Milosevic A. The use of porcelain veneers to restore palatal tooth loss. *Restor Dent* 1990; **6**: 15-18.

12 McLundie A C. Localised palatal tooth surface loss and its treatment with porcelain laminates. *Restor Dent* **7**: 43-44.

13 Crawford P J M, Aboush Y E Y. The use of adhesively retained gold onlays in the management of dental erosion in a child: a 4-year case report. *Br Dent J* 1993; **175**: 414-416.

14 Rawlinson A, Winstanley R B. The management of severe dental erosion using posterior occlusal porcelain veneers and an anterior overdenture. *Restor Dent* 1988; **4**: 10-16.

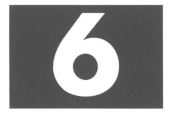

Prevention and maintenance

J. L. Wickens[1]

Awareness of tooth surface loss has increased among both dentists and patients. This is, no doubt, because of the decline in caries rate and the control of periodontal disease with the result that many more people remain partially or fully dentate into old age.[1] The media have also been influential in raising patients' awareness of appearance. These factors have led to a shift in patients' demands and a change in the practice of dentistry.[2]

Caries and periodontal disease can be controlled with appropriate education and professional support even in the older patient. In contrast, the dental profession does not seem to have reached a consensus on the action needed in cases of tooth surface loss. This current series of articles has brought together many views on this topic. They all have one recurrent theme; that prevention of tooth surface loss is preferable to restoration. The latter will often be extensive, expensive and carries with it a lifetime commitment to maintenance and further restorative procedures.

Effective prevention must involve:
• Patient education
• Early recognition
• Use of predictors
• Control of further tooth surface loss.

Prevention requires an understanding of the aetiology and recognition of early signs and symptoms.[3] Tooth surface loss often has a complex character making it difficult to determine the aetiological factors responsible for dental wear. This combined with non-specific signs and symptoms has resulted in a slow appreciation of the disease patterns by the profession and patients. The consequences are that recognition is often so late that prevention alone is inappropriate.

Terminology tends to confuse the issue further; terms in current use do not follow the common dental pattern of describing the physical characteristics of the condition. Rather all refer to the possible cause (erosion, abrasion, attrition and, more recently, abfraction) and it follows that care may be directed at a sole attributed aetiological factor, disregarding the common multi-factorial nature of the condition. The description of the physical effect, ie 'tooth surface loss' or 'tooth wear', encourages a broader perspective. This results in less confusion over classification, accepting that both preventive measures and treatment have common

ground independent of the dominant attributable cause.[4]

Prevention also includes the identification of those individuals who may be at risk. There are indicators that may be helpful. Tooth surface loss may begin in the primary dentition. For a given individual, there is evidence of a link between this and tooth surface loss in the permanent dentition. Nystrom *et al.*[5] found that horizontal wear of the maxillary anterior teeth at 14 years of age, predicted well the continuing wear of these teeth at 18 years of age. Maximal anterior bite force, intake of low pH foodstuffs and a low gonial angle correlated well with the total wear area on the anterior teeth. These features, along with the knowledge that the number and distribution of teeth with occlusal wear increase with age,[6] would imply that once wear begins, it is ongoing at a steady pace. The literature, though, does not support this. Tooth surface loss can occur in 'bouts' as habits and morphological and psychological states change. For instance, Cash found that bruxism in children generally increases with age through the mixed dentition and then decreases.[7] A further complication is that while the dominant aetiological factor may have diminished, the tooth will have been altered to render it more susceptible to other factors in tooth wear, such as erosion due to dietary acids. The diagnosis is thus complex and further highlights the need for comprehensive and broadbased patient education.

Communication is also important in prevention of advanced tooth wear. Careful questioning regarding patients' dietary, gastric or parafunctional habits may indicate the reasons for the state of the dentition. Adults who report parafunctional activity are known to have more incisal and occlusal tooth surface loss than those unaware of a grinding habit.[8] It has been suggested that tooth grinding is a motor disturbance that is not limited to the masticatory muscles but also manifests itself as generally increased body movement.[9] Two aetiological models have been developed, the structural model based on the role played by malocclusion or alterations in maxillo-mandibular relations, while a functional model highlights the role of stress, emotional tension and personality characteristics.[10] However, there is no 'cause and effect' relationship established in longitudinal studies to give any predictive value to either of them.

Therefore, the following groups should be

Effective maintenance is necessary to minimise further tooth wear and control other dental disease. Restorative dentistry provided without such control is frequently unsuccessful.

[1]*Consultant in Restorative Dentistry, Eastman Dental Hospital and Honorary Senior Lecturer, Eastman Dental Institute for Oral Health Care Sciences, University of London, 256 Gray's Inn Road WC1X 8LD*

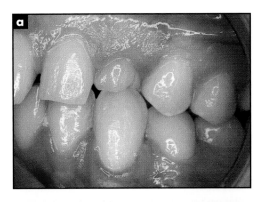

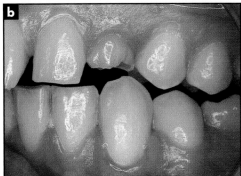

Fig. 1a and 1b The localised effects of retaining a primary tooth

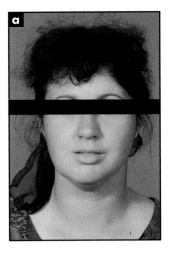

Fig. 2a to 2d Tooth wear presenting as a case of gross facial asymmetry

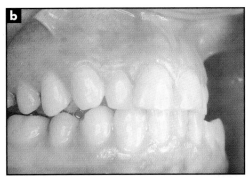

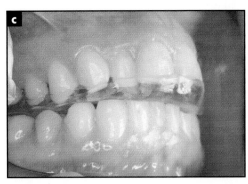

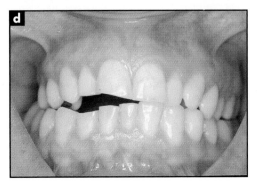

considered at greater risk of tooth surface loss. Those with a history of:

- Tooth surface loss as a child
- Reported parafunctional activity
- Heavy anterior bite force, possibly related to a low gonial angle
- Eating disorders, including the excessive intake of low pH beverages
- Medical disorders resulting in gastric reflux or voluntary vomiting.

The ability to use such information depends on the patient reporting aspects of their own behaviour which they may not consider relevant to their dental problems. Thus the teeth themselves may provide the first indication of an abnormal habit or disease. Bartlett recently highlighted this when he showed that 17 of the 26 patients presenting with tooth surface loss on the palatal aspect of their upper anterior teeth had unreported or undiagnosed daytime gastro-oesophageal reflux.[11] This illustrates one of the fundamental difficulties in predicting tooth surface loss.

Why prevent tooth surface loss?

The effects of tooth surface loss are frequently not limited simply to wear of the teeth. It will also affect the surrounding structures. Teeth try to maintain functional contact, both occlusally and interproximally,[12] and tend to move as they wear. Alveolar bone and the periodontal complex move with the tooth, such that the congruity of the gingival margin will often indicate where there has been tooth movement. Figure 1 shows the localised effect of retaining an increasingly worn primary tooth, with the result that the opposing and adjacent teeth have encroached on the space required for an aesthetic or functional replacement. Treatment for this adult has been complicated by a lack of earlier management of tooth wear.

Wear caused by parafunctional activity is frequently accompanied by compensatory changes in the dentition that allow occlusal contacts and function to be maintained.

Tooth wear in the anterior segment of the mouth is often unsightly, driving the patient to seek dental advice. It will very commonly have been accompanied by changes in the occlusal relationships which may have functional implications and complicate restorative procedures. Attempts are frequently made to meet the aesthetic demands of patients without due consideration of the functional aspects of worn teeth. This can result in either failure of the restorations or wear of the opposing teeth due to inappropriate loading.

Patients may seek help only when gross changes, such as facial asymmetry (fig. 2), have taken place . Investigation of the patient's maxillo-mandibular relationship in the retruded axis position revealed an underlying skeletal discrepancy of the dental bases producing an edge-to-edge tooth relationship. A functional 'best fit' had been assumed and tooth wear had resulted from parafunctional activity in this position. Earlier recognition would perhaps have prevented compensatory tooth movement and simplified corrective treatment.

Prevention of further tooth wear ideally involves elimination of the causative agent but this simple action is often impossible. A preventive regime with features common to all cases can be developed which aims to modify habits and protect the remaining tooth structure. This should include:
- Patient education
- Dietary and toothbrushing advice (technique and timing of brushing)
- Fluoride (patient and/or professional application) dentifrice and mouthwash
- Careful monitoring of tooth structure (serial casts, photos and the use of indices).[13]

Further actions may be prescribed that are specific to the dominant aetiological factor.
- Parafunctional activity, constant or phasic in nature, will demand the provision of a protective occlusal splint. Details of these appliances were given in Part 3.
- An integrated approach with medical colleagues is recommended in cases of voluntary vomiting and suspected gastro-oesophageal reflux.[14]

Figure 3 shows the serial casts of a young lady produced for her in 1978, 1988 and 1995. The casts allow a much clearer assessment of the extent of wear than would have been evident from an intra-oral examination. This technique, which is used insufficiently frequently, provides valuable evidence for judging the extent and pace of tooth wear, the success of preventive measures and the need for restorative treatment to protect the remaining tooth structure.

The timing of restorative intervention can be problematical. The conservative placement of plastic restorative materials in erosion lesions (fig. 4) may be considered part of preventive care. In areas not susceptible to high loads, they have an excellent retention rate.[15] Signs and symptoms from the teeth may indicate a need for restorations but may also solely be evidence of active tooth surface loss. However, the dentist must be alert to wear which causes no symptoms and ensure that preventive regimes are established. Successful prevention, though, will be dependent on an appreciation by the patient of the long-term benefits of such regimes. A team approach, using the hygienist to reinforce the modification in habits, will assist with this difficult task of sustained motivation. Without intervention, the number and distribution of teeth with incisal and occlusal wear will increase with age.[6]

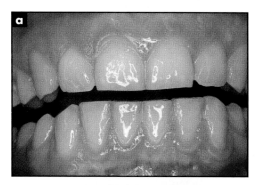
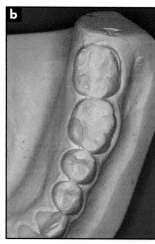
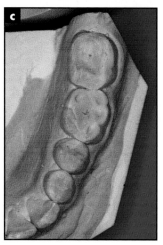
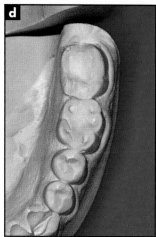
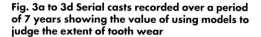

Fig. 3a to 3d Serial casts recorded over a period of 7 years showing the value of using models to judge the extent of tooth wear

The indications for proceeding from 'prevention' to 'intervention' with restorations are:
- Symptoms and signs associated with the tooth surface loss that cannot be controlled through preventive regimes. These not only include pain and sensitivity but also a deterioration in the appearance of the teeth.
- The remaining tooth structure requires protection. When failure to restore may lead to the loss of the tooth or render later restoration much more complicated.

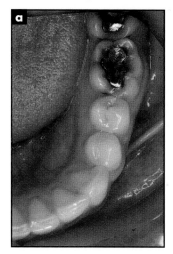
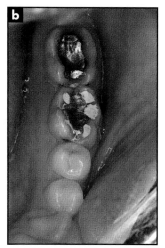

Fig. 4a and 4b The placement of plastic restorations in erosion lesions may be considered as a part of preventive care

Restoration of teeth with worn functional surfaces, presents three main difficulties:

1 The functional relationship of the teeth will have changed. The occlusal table is widened bringing a broader aspect of the tooth into function, generating broad, flat occlusal contacts which lack stability. This was discussed in detail in Part 3 of the series.

2 Clinical crown height is reduced. Retention and resistance form for conventional crown preparation will be compromised following adequate tooth removal to provide space for the restorative material.

3 The quality of the tooth structure, with exposure of large areas of dentine, may limit the use of desirable, conservative adhesive techniques.

Maintenance of patients with restored dentitions is necessary to prevent the prevention of further damage

The aim is to maintain stability in the oral environment, given that the original aetiological factors are often incompletely controlled. A maintenance regime should have the following characteristics:

• Development of an individual programme at the outset of treatment
• Use a team approach to ensure compliance
• Consider all patients to be 'high risk'
• Consider providing a protective occlusal splint for nocturnal wear after restoration.

Maintenance is an aspect of care that is commonly overlooked but cannot be overstressed. The regime devised for a patient will be influenced by the degree of control of the

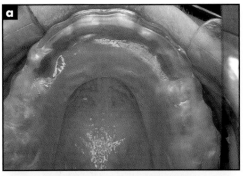

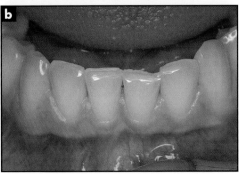

Fig. 5a and 5b Splint therapy used in a case of suspected parafunctional activity

aetiological factors that resulted in the original tooth wear and by information gained from literature and clinical practice on the past performance of restorations in similar circumstances.

Control of the aetiological factors

Human nature ensures that a patient complies with requests to modify their habits for usually only a limited period while under professional review. Reviews should therefore be at intervals that are sufficiently short to keep the patient motivated. These need to be appropriate for the individual patient and the whole dental team should participate. It is unlikely that all the aetiological factors causing the tooth wear will have been identified and controlled. For example, patients who demonstrated parafunctional activity at the time of initial presentation should wear an occlusal splint post-restoratively. In figure 5. the worn palatal surfaces of the upper anterior teeth in this teenager had been protected with adhesively retained metal backings. Both the patient and clinician were concerned that the lower anterior teeth would be at risk of further wear; she was provided with a set of base-line casts and a hard acrylic maxillary guard for night use. An annual recall programme has been considered appropriate for her. The dentist/hygienist team is extremely important in the recall strategy; the hygienist may see the patient more regularly and can alert the dentist to obvious lesions, changes in tooth contour and concerns expressed by the patient.

The survival of restorations in the oral environment has been widely investigated. Most commonly the performance of the restorative material has been assessed and this is often unrelated to the environment in which it was employed. For instance, secondary caries and marginal degradation are cited as the two most common reasons for failure of restorations.[16] Precipitating factors such as facets, a lack of clinical crown height or the substrate used for bonding restorations, have not been evaluated. The literature indicates that amalgam remains the material of choice for routine posterior restorations and gold for more extensive ones; composite materials should be limited to small restorations with limited occlusal loading,[17] mainly to satisfy patients' cosmetic demands.

Secondary caries, post-operative sensitivity, fracture and poor anatomical form are common reasons for failure of large posterior composites. Worn dentitions are frequently patched and repaired with adhesively retained resins as the defects often do not lend themselves to conventional cavity preparation for amalgam. Deterioration and failure of such restorations can contribute to a loss of occlusal stability which is added to by continued wear of the teeth.

Figure 6 shows a worn dentition that has been restored with indirect restorations in the

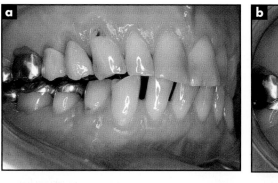
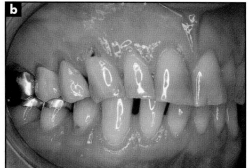
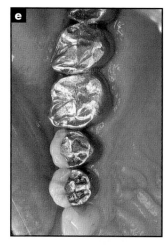
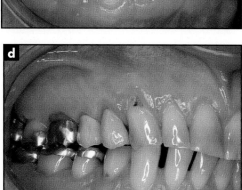
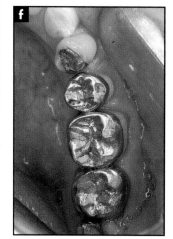

Fig. 6a to 6f A worn dentition restored with indirect restorations in the posterior quadrants

posterior quadrants. The occlusal environment at that time provided appropriate anterior guidance with posterior disclusion. While a maxillary hard acrylic guard was provided post-restoratively for night use, by the patient's own admission compliance was poor. The result has been continued wear of the canine teeth, with shallowing the anterior guidance to such an extent that the posterior teeth are in contact throughout lateral excursive movements. The gold restorations have become worn and occlusal stability has been lost. This expensive restorative procedure has been undermined by lack of compliance with preventive regimes. It highlights the care needed in matching restorative treatment plans with the needs, wishes and abilities of the patient. Patient involvement in the planning of care must be comprehensive and the definitive treatment plan not made before a thorough period of evaluation has been completed.

The recall appointment

The routine at these visits should be:
• Listen
• Look
• Learn!

Listen — general conversation with the patient may indicate whether the original aetiological factors in the tooth wear are under control. It is also important to consider the patient's views; for example if they think that their splint is a social barrier, it may not be worn regularly. Major life events may also affect the ability to carry out normal daily routines.

Look — intra-oral examination may support

aspects of the history. Comparison of the current situation with the original set of casts is imperative (fig. 3). These casts should be the property and responsibility of the patient. This encourages a degree of 'ownership' and hopefully improves the patient's interest in their condition. Indices for monitoring tooth wear have been proposed by a number of authors and were discussed briefly in the first article in this series. These may be helpful but the dynamic nature of the consequences of tooth wear still makes assessment difficult.

Monitoring tooth surface loss is demanding: frequency of re-evaluation must be appropriate, not only to monitor preventive regimes, but also to be able to judge the need for and timing of restoration. Once restored, further complications can arise. Marginal deficiencies related to all indirectly fabricated restorations are filled at cementation with soluble, permeable cements, whether of acid-base or resin variety. Detection of marginal gaps is often very difficult, especially when margins are inaccessible.[18] Their assessment is based on tactile acuity alone rather than being supported by visual inspection, as with supra-gingival margins. Radiographs provide an invaluable adjunct to this inspection.

In well controlled cases, biological failures through caries and periodontal disease will be rare but continued wear of tooth or restoration may still occur. There remains considerable difficulty in controlling a disease with a multi-factorial aetiology and varying predominant features.

Symptoms to be addressed at recall in relation to continuing wear are:

tooth surface loss

1 Department of Health. *An oral health strategy for England.* London; Department of Health, 1994.

2 *Dental Practice Board 1994-1995 annual report.* Eastbourne, 1995.

3 Milosevic A. Tooth wear: an aetiological and diagnostic problem. *EurJ Prosthodont Rest Dent* 1993; **1**: 173-178.

4 Bader J, Levitch L, Shugars D, Heymann H, McClure F. How dentists classified and treated non carious cervical lesions. *J Am Dent Assoc* 1993; **124**: 46.

5 Nystrom M, Kononen M, Alaluusua S, Evalahti M, Vartiovaara J. Development of horizontal tooth wear in maxillary anterior teeth from five to eighteen years of age. *J Dent Res* 1990; **69**:1765-1770.

6 Hugoson A, Bergendal T, Ekfeldt A, Helkimo M. Prevalence and severity of incisal and occlusal tooth wear in an adult Swedish population. *Acta Odontol Scand* 1988; **46**: 255 - 265.

7 Cash R. Bruxism in children: a review of the literature. *J Pedodont* 1988; **12**: 107-127.

8 Ekfeldt A, Hugoson A, Bergendal T, Helkimo M. An individual tooth wear index and an analysis of factors correlated to incisal and occlusal tooth wear in an adult Swedish population. *Acta Odontol Scand* 1990; **48**: 344-349.

9 Sjoholm T, Polo O, Alihanka A. Sleep movement in tooth grinders. *J Craniomandib Disorders* 1992; **6**: 184-191.

10 Biondi M, Picardi A. Temperomandibular joint pain dysfunction syndrome and bruxism: etiopathogenesis and treatment from a psychosomatic integrative point of view. *Psychotherapy & Psychosomatic* 1993; **59**: 84-98.

11 Bartlett D, Evans D, Smith B. Simultaneous oral and oesophageal pH measurement after a reflux provoking meal. *J Dent Res* 1994; Spec Issue Abst 70.

12 Love W, Adams R. Tooth movement into edentulous areas. *J Prosthet Dent* 1971; **25**: 271-278.

13 Smith B, Knight J. An index for measuring the wear of teeth. *Br Dent J* 1984; **156**: 435-438.

14 Cowan R, Sabates C, Gross K, EllledgeD. Integrating dental & medical care for a chronic bulimia nervosa patient: a case report. *Quintessence Int* 1991; **22**: 553-557.

15 Brandau H E, Ziemiecki T L, Charbeneau G T. Restoration of cervical contours on nonprepared teeth using glass ionomer cement: a 4 fi year report. *J Am Dent Assoc* 1984; **108**: 782-783.

16 Rykke M. Dental materials for posterior restorations. *Endod Dent Traumatol* 1992; **8**: 139-148.

17 Lundin S. Studies on posterior composite resins with special reference to Class II restorations. *Swedish Dent J* 1990; **73** (supplement).

18 Christenson G. Marginal fit of gold inlay castings. *J Prosthet Dent* 1966; **16**: 297-395.

19 Chadwick B, Dummer P. Factors affecting the diagnostic quality of bitewing radiographs: a review. *Br Dent J* 1998; **184**: 80-84.

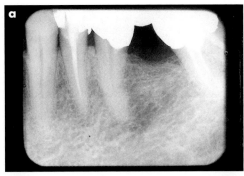

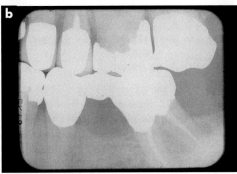

Fig. 7a A long cone radiograph of tooth 5̅ (35) apparently showing a distal cavity; Fig. 7b A bite wing radiograph of the same tooth confirming the clinical finding of sound tissue

• Pain/sensitivity possibly indicating that tooth surface loss is occurring faster than any reparative mechanisms
• Sharp edges of tooth or restoration
• Fracture of tooth or restorative material
• Facets on tooth or restorative material.

Sensitivity and sharp edges are commonly symptoms of rapid erosion, whereas fracture and facets are often indicators of continuing parafunctional activity. Unfortunately, the presence of these features is not always consistent and therefore serve only as potential indicators of the predominant aetiological factor.

Radiographs

The frequency with which these are taken and the views used are, once again, influenced by features of the specific case. Frequency will relate to the perceived stability of the situation and the possible value to be gained from them. An average interval between radiographs would be 6 to 24 months but they can be taken at any interval when they will aid either in monitoring or diagnosis.

The view taken must be appropriate:
• Bitewings: these will give information on the integrity of the tooth, restoration margins, and bone levels in the inter-proximal region.
• Long cone periapicals taken using a paralleling technique : these provide periapical information but have poorer definition of interproximal features at coronal level, eg caries.

Accurate and repeatable views aid diagnosis. These can only be obtained using a holder which supports the film and guides the radiographic beam.[19]

• Orthopantomogram: this provides a general view of the teeth and jaws but is generally of little use for specific tooth-related dental diagnoses.

When a tooth has been restored, diagnosis of a carious lesion from a radiograph can be very difficult, particularly where there are no clinical signs or symptoms. Radiographs can be misleading and a diagnosis must be made from compound clinical and radiographic information. Figure 7a shows a long cone radiograph of tooth 5̅ (35) restored with a gold cast retainer many years previously. There were no symptoms from this tooth. There appeared to be distal cervical caries, however, no clinical evidence for this could be found. A bitewing view (fig. 7b) showed the suspicious appearance on the original long cone periapical was a shadow.

Radiographs form a valuable diagnostic aid in the maintenance programme. The views taken and the interval between radiographs should be selected on the basis of the clinical benefit that will be derived.

This paper has described the features of an effective maintenance programme. It comes in this series before papers which describe restorative intervention. This reflects the importance of the topic. Where the maintenance programme is ineffective, the restorative work defective or simply worn out, failure becomes more likely. The next paper will describe how such failures should be managed and ways in which their impact can be lessened.

This article is based on a presentation at The Medical Society of London on 10 May 1995 as part of the Alpha Omega lecture programme.

7 Dealing with failures

J. L. Wickens[1]

Previous articles in this series have discussed some of the consequences of tooth surface loss. These can necessitate the restoration of teeth. Part 6 discussed the importance of establishing effective maintenance for patients if further dental disease were to be minimised. However, once teeth have been restored, there is the possibility that those restorations will fail: there is in fact a certainty that that they will do so. This can be either through recurrent dental disease or as a result of their age, they simply just wear out. Consequently, managing failure is an everyday part of being a dentist.

Effective maintenance will prolong the life of restorations. This requires that the dentist is vigilant and alert to early signs of failure while monitoring the slow but inevitable deterioration in ageing crowns and fillings.

Intervention becomes necessary when:
• Signs or symptoms from the teeth are unacceptable to the patient
• The situation created by the failure is detrimental to the stability of the dentition.

The dental literature is not particularly helpful in describing the factors that influence the lifespan of crowns and bridges. Of those that are available, one indicates that certain types of bridge retainer are more likely to fail than others.[1] Limited amounts of more specific information are available: bridges with three or more abutments have a greater chance of failure than those with two or less.[2] Good, in a retrospective study, showed the mean survival time of an indirect restoration placed in the Conservation Department at the Eastman Dental Hospital to be over 20 years.[3] However, the lack of criteria for placement of the restorations makes such data of limited application. Assessment of a very large number of restorations in a prospective study will be required before conclusions can be drawn regarding the intra-oral factors which affect their lifespan.

It has long been suspected, but only recently shown, that precluding coronal leakage is important to endodontic success. Similarly, it is accepted but unproven that the prognosis for a restoration is influenced by the way in which loads on the tooth or restoration are distributed. Lateral loads, such as those created in the posterior dentition by non-working side interferences, may cause fracture or loss of cementation. Supporting this, Hojjatie and Anusavice have suggested from their study on glass ceramic crowns that failure of these restorations is more influenced by the orientation of the applied load than the occlusal thickness of the material.[4] Structural integrity remains important, but the environment into which a restoration is placed must be considered. This is particularly important for those who exert high occlusal loads through parafunctional activity. When the predominant factor is erosion, failure is likely to be due to continued erosion of the tooth or cement lute undermining the margins of the existing restoration. This results in a loss of marginal integrity and ultimately failure as a result of secondary caries.

Dental caries is the most frequently described cause of failure of restorations. However, this view is probably simplistic. For example, the stresses applied to the cement film retaining a crown may in the end cause the lute to begin to disintegrate. This allows leakage and eventually dental caries may develop. The primary cause of failure is not the decay but the factors that caused the cement to disintegrate. Diagnosing the cause of a failure is frequently not easy and a logical sequence for analysing the problem is helpful.

Dealing with failures

Where failure has occurred:
• Establish the likely cause
• Deal with symptoms (pain, mobility, unacceptable appearance etc)
• Assess and, if indicated, modify the occlusal environment
• Assess and protect the remaining tooth structure
• Plan future restoration
• Provide the restoration
• Prevent further damage through preventive regimes.

Figure 1 shows a failed complex bridge with secondary caries and periapical pathology associated with the retainers. To deal with these problems, the sequence described above was followed. This bridge was of complex design with multiple, rigidly-linked retainers and the cement lute had been stressed and failed. A simpler design would be advocated if the bridge were to be remade. The bridge was removed, the remaining tooth structure evaluated and the bridge relined and replaced as a temporary measure. Reparative dental treatment and future planning could then be undertaken in a controlled environment.

> **Managing failures requires an understanding of their causes. These vary and each failure must be analysed if a further restoration is to have a reasonable prospect of success.**

[1]Consultant in Restorative Dentistry, Eastman Dental Hospital and Honorary Senior Lecturer, Eastman Dental Institute for Oral Health Care Sciences, University of London, 256 Gray's Inn Road WC1X 8LD

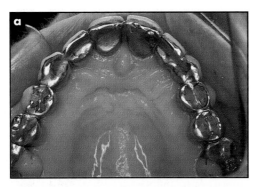

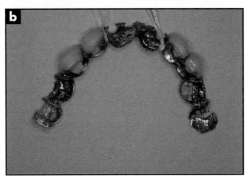

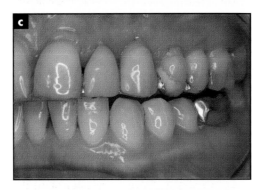

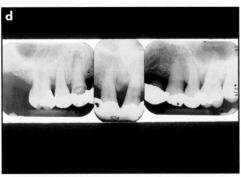

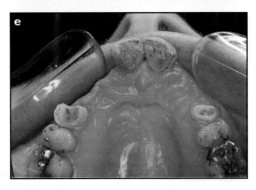

Fig. 1a to 1e Failure of a complex bridge with secondary caries and periapical pathology associated with the abutment teeth

Active caries or periodontal disease indicates that the maintenance programme developed for that patient must be reconsidered. All teeth should be carefully evaluated. In many cases of tooth wear there will have been considerable loss of clinical crown prior to restoration. This will have compromised the retention and resistance form of the preparations for the cast restorations or the bonding area for adhesive ones. Therefore care should be taken, not only in treating the presenting problem, but concurrently evaluating the other restored teeth. The occlusal examination is important in making a diagnosis and in helping to avoid a further failure. The following is a summary of the features of this part of the examination:

- Check occlusal stability and note any changes such as recent loss of teeth, further wear or replacement of restorations which may have affected its stability.
- Look for facets on the opposing dentition
- Check all excursive pathways of mandibular movement and ascertain whether there was adequate space for the restoration. If not, it may be an indication that it was an interference. An interference may often be removed by modification of the preparation or the opposing tooth. Where it was a guidance surface, consideration should be given to distributing these loads more widely. These adjustments are, however, best planned on a set of articulated study casts prior to execution in the mouth. Only those that can be accomplished simply and predictably should be executed without extra-oral planning. The original crown may be recemented or a new temporary crown provided. This temporary restoration will permit full assessment of the appropriate functional form prior to remaking the crown.

Failure resulting in loss of either an adhesive or a conventional restoration, which covered the functional surface, may have permitted overeruption of the tooth itself or its antagonist. Repreparation of the tooth is the obvious method to re-create the space, however tooth structure was in short supply to begin with. Localised intrusion of the prepared tooth may be a better option but caution should be exercised not to disturb an otherwise stable occlusion. Strategies for creating space for restorations have been discussed briefly in earlier articles and will be described more fully in future ones.

Material selection

Failures can be 'mechanical'. Rapid failure of a restoration usually indicates an inappropriate choice of a material for that situation; for instance, the use of materials which are primarily dependent on enamel bonding employed in sites mainly composed of dentine. The risk is greatest when the material has been used in thin section or when the loading is high. Clearly, in these circumstances, material selection should be reconsidered. While technological advances in dentinal adhesion are rapid, the substrate to which there is a lower adhesive bond will dominate the overall bond strength once it occupies more than half of the bonding surface.[5]

Most materials have an optimal range of thickness for successful use. McLean recommends porcelain to be at least 1 mm but not more than 2 mm thick in functional areas.[6] Limited clinical crown height in the worn dentition often precludes the predictable use of this material.

A common site for failure of many materials is at an interface, either between it and the tooth or between two restorative materials as in a porcelain-fused-to-metal crown. Load at an interface should be avoided. Prior to replacing a failed restoration, the occlusal contacts should be examined and assessed. Ideally, any junction or margin should lie at least 1 mm from the intercuspal contact. Where the restorative material is involved in excursive movements, it must be well supported. This applies to any restorative material, but is particularly pertinent to brittle materials such as porcelain, amalgam and heavily-filled composite resin.

Failure may be caused by poor technical work, the responsibility for which lies ultimately with the clinician. Figure 2 clearly shows that the best efforts of the clinician to ensure retention of this bridge have not been matched by the technical quality as the axial grooves in the preparation have not been reproduced in the final casting.

Aesthetic failure

One of the most common failures to be found in restored worn teeth is in the appearance of the final restorations. This is because of the changes in position of the teeth and soft tissues that have taken place as the teeth have worn. The relationship between the tooth and gingival margin has often been maintained while the teeth have migrated to maintain contact with their opponents. This keeps the incisal edges not far short of their original position. As part of restoration, the teeth need to be lengthened both incisally and gingivally to produce an aesthetic result. If this is not recognised at the outset, the final restorations will reflect the original worn teeth and appear a little longer. Proportions can only be altered by crown lengthening or reorganisation of the occlusal relationship. The principles underlying surgical crown lengthening procedures are described later in the series. Diagnostic waxing is invaluable in preventing this type of failure; it not only aids the clinician but involves patients in their treatment. It also often helps to explain the many limitations that exist in achieving an ideal aesthetic result.

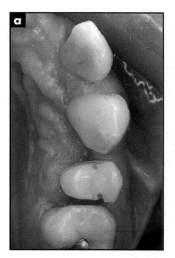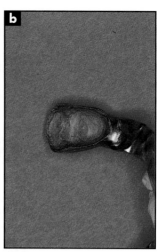

Fig. 2a and 2b Poor technical quality as the prime reason for failure of a bridge

Repair of restorations

Repair of restorations, if possible, is cost effective and improves their longevity.[7] Where repair is contemplated, the cause of the failure must be determined so that the restoration is altered such that whatever pre-disposed to the failure is eliminated. For example, if the isthmus of an MOD amalgam restoration fractures it is a sign that there was insufficient bulk of amalgam. If only one half of the restoration is to be replaced, either the isthmus should be deepened or the opposing tooth contacts inspected and if appropriate adjusted before the repair to the MOD is made.

Caries associated with the margin of a crown does not always demand replacement of the restoration. If a repair is to be made, restorative principles should not be ignored. A sufficiently large window must be prepared in the marginal area of the crown to allow straight line access to the dental caries. Only by using such an approach can all the caries be eliminated while also creating room for a reasonable bulk of restorative material.

Provision for failure

Dental restorations have a finite 'life span'. The reduced quantity and quality of the remaining tooth structure and poor control of aetiological factors complicate the selection of suitable restorative materials. Many patients with worn teeth are young and consideration must be given to the potential need for further restorations during their lifetime. Techniques and materials that permit conservation of tooth structure should be selected where possible. Adhesive techniques of the type described in Part 5 of this series have much to commend them in patients with worn teeth. Restorative procedures can be less involved than for more conventional methods. Future provision is facilitated by preserving tooth structure, while damage to the dental pulp through extensive tooth preparation will also be

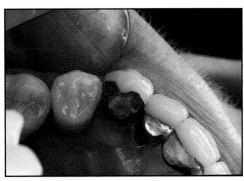

Fig. 3 The provision of a 'sleeping slot' to provide provision against failure in an abutment tooth

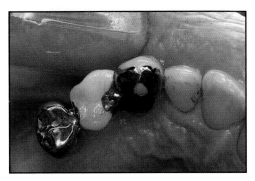

Fig. 4 Rest seats and guide planes for future provision of a partial denture

There are instances when several units are at risk of early failure and the remaining teeth will not support further fixed restorations. Teeth that have a better prognosis should be targeted and restorations designed with guide planes and rest seats to accept a partial denture in the future (fig. 4) should this prove necessary. This allows for cost-effective tooth replacement even if alternative means, such as implants, were to be considered later.

This paper and the previous one have promoted the concept that restorations will behave predictably if they are provided to a high standard and in a controlled environment. The occlusion, either natural or restored, must therefore be as stable as possible and prevention of wear is very important. Laboratory techniques can be practised that seek to anticipate changes in the occlusion, for example canine guidance gradually wearing into group function. Such a considered approach is commendable but its success cannot be guaranteed. Predicting the changes in the relationship of teeth is virtually impossible and there can be no substitute for careful monitoring and taking action where indicated.

In contrast to the disease processes of caries and periodontal disease, a professional consensus has not yet been reached on the control, or action needed, in cases of tooth surface loss. This is in part because until comparatively recently it has not been considered to be a widespread problem, for example the Adult Dental Health Report of 1988 did not include it. This does perhaps indicate how quickly it has sprung to prominence.

Restoration of short teeth can present difficulties such as compromised resistance form for indirect restorations and a lack of bulk of restorative material for directly-placed ones. The inherent lack of stability of wearing dentitions is likely to increase the loads on what can be compromised restorations. It is not therefore surprising that restorative failures are frequently seen where restorations are placed under such conditions. This paper has discussed how such failures may best be managed.

This paper introduced the role that adhesive dentistry can play in the management of tooth surface loss. Worn teeth have become more common in children and adolescents and present particular preventive and restorative difficulties. The next article in the series looks at tooth surface loss in the young patient and describes the use of adhesive dental materials.

This article is based on a presentation at The Medical Society of London on 10 May 1995 as part of the Alpha Omega lecture programme.

1 Roberts D. The failure of retainers in bridge prostheses. An analysis of 2000 retainers. *Br Dent J* 1970; **128**: 117-124.

2 Foster L. Failed conventional bridgework from general dental practice: clinical aspects and treatment needs of 142 cases. *Br Dent J* 1990; **168**: 199-201.

3 Good J. *Survival analysis of indirect restorations in extensively restored dentitions.* London: Eastman Dental Institute for Oral Health Care Sciences, University of London.1996, MSc report.

4 Anusavice K J, Hojjatie B. Tensile stress in glass-ceramic crowns: effect of flaws and cement voids. *Int J Prosthodontics* 1992; **5**: 351-358.

5 Aboush Y, Jenkins C. The bonding of an adhesive resin cement to single and combined adherends encountered in resin-bonded bridgework: an in vitro study. *Br Dent J* 1991; **171**: 166.

6 McLean J. *Science and art of dental ceramics.* Vol 1. London: Quintessence, 1979.

7 Mjor I A. Repair and replacement of failed restorations. *Int Dent J* 1993; **43**: 466-472.

avoided. The relationship with the patient is built on trust; this cannot involve impractical concepts of maintenance. Patients should be part of the decisions made in treatment planning so that the risks of restorative procedures are appreciated and the consequences of adverse outcomes minimised. One method used to minimise the impact of failures is to incorporate 'provision for failure' into restorations. Features can be built in to facilitate continuity of care with minimal disruption to other teeth should failure occur.

In older and more extensively restored dentitions where disease experience has been greatest, loss of the most compromised teeth can sometimes be anticipated. Restorations on the teeth which have a better prognosis should, whenever possible, be designed to allow a change from being a single unit to a retainer for a bridge or partial denture. The aim is to avoid the fabrication of new restorations when a tooth is lost. The most common example of 'provision for failure' is the incorporation of a 'sleeping female' in the distal aspect of a crown which might be a potential retainer (fig. 3). For example, if 3|(13), 4|(14) and 5|(15) were crowned but 4|(14) were restored with a post crown, it would be appropriate to consider a 'sleeping slot' in the distal of 3|(13). This allows conservation of the intact mesial retainer were 4|(14) to be lost.

8 Tooth wear in the child and the youth

K. Harley[1]

The previous articles in this series have discussed tooth surface loss in the adult. Dentists will be aware of this problem in younger patients where it can sometimes cause very severe damage at an early stage in life. The management of the child and adolescent has a number of similarities to adults with a need for effective prevention. When restoration becomes necessary, consideration must be given to lifelong management of the patient and adhesive techniques have a major role to play.

Tooth wear has become a major clinical challenge for dentists treating the young patient today. Although this wear is undoubtedly due to a combination of erosion, abrasion and attrition, the major factor in this age-group is erosion. The evidence that the prevalence of erosion is increasing remains largely anecdotal. However fewer dentists are questioning this as they see the problem growing in their own working environment. It has still to be demonstrated whether the prevalence is actually increasing or the heightened awareness of this problem is simply a matter of improved recognition and reporting. It is interesting to note that as early as 1908 G V Black stated that although erosion is rare compared with caries, once a practitioner is aware of erosion he will actually see it in many more patients:[1] a philosophy which is not out of place today. It remains a challenge for paediatric dentists familiar with the early diagnosis of erosion to teach their colleagues how to recognise the problem before it is too late. The first important study that attempted to determine the prevalence of dental erosion in children was the UK Child Dental Health Survey of 1993.[2] It was reported that 52% of 5-year-olds had erosion of their primary incisors with 25% showing dentinal or pulpal involvement. Of 11–14-year-olds, 28% were found to have erosion of their upper incisors. The higher susceptibility of the primary dentition is thought to be due to a reduced thickness of the enamel and its greater solubility in acid.

Aetiology

All acids, whether intrinsic or extrinsic in origin, are capable of causing erosion. While gastric acid cannot be discounted the overwhelming evidence would suggest that the primary aetiology in this age group is the consumption of fruit juices, squashes and carbonated beverages. Data supplied by the Soft Drinks manufacturers showing a seven-fold increase in the consumption of soft drinks between 1950 and 1990 support this.[3] Soft drink intake is much higher in younger age-groups. They have been reported to provide as much as one-fifth of added sugars in the diet of 11–12 year old children and 42% of fruit drinks are consumed by children aged between 2 and 9 years.[4] Nutritionists and dieticians are increasingly concerned that children are not eating sufficient quantities of food to maintain the correct calorific intake and level of nutrients for growth and development because they fill up on large quantities of fruit-based drinks. Of equal concern is the evidence that eating patterns established in childhood persist into adulthood. Children with erosion of the primary dentition have already established patterns of eating and drinking which place them in a high risk group for damage to the permanent dentition. In 1995 it was projected that by the year 2000, 12–15-year-olds would be drinking 50% more soft drinks.[5] The earlier such behaviour can be modified the better for the teeth.

Erosion is not linked simply to a high intake of acidic beverages but also to the frequency, the method and the timing of consumption. The latter is particularly important with respect to mealtimes and prior to toothbrushing. Erosion may be exacerbated by high standards of oral hygiene. Where a bedtime drink precedes bedtime toothbrushing, the potential for an even greater loss of tooth substance can exist.[6]

The development of dental erosion in an individual is dependent on a number of additional factors. Some of these are inherent to that person and cannot be altered by dietary management. Examples are the buffering capacity of saliva, the solubility of the tooth structure in acid and the relationship between the hard and soft tissues. The overall consumption of acidic foodstuffs in addition to beverages is also important as is the general health of the child or adolescent. A recent study to investigate the relationship between dental erosion and gastro-oesophageal reflux (GOR) found that only 9 of 53 affected children examined between 2 and 16 years, showed any signs of dental erosion and of these only one had erosion involving dentine.[7] The authors concluded that dental erosion may not be as great a problem in children with GOR as some authorities believe it to be in adults.

Tooth surface loss is an increasing problem in younger individuals. Preventive strategies are essential while adhesive dentistry should be used whenever possible if restoration is necessary.

[1]Consultant and Honorary Senior Lecturer, Department of Pediatric Dentistry, Eastman Dental Hospital, University College London Hopitals Trust and the Eastman Dental Institute for Oral Health Care Sciences, University of London, 256 Gray's Inn Road, London WC1 8LD

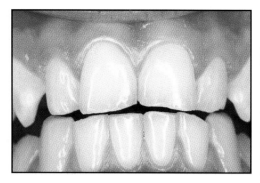

Fig. 1 A loss of surface anatomy

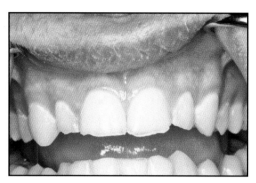

Fig. 2 Increased incisal translucency

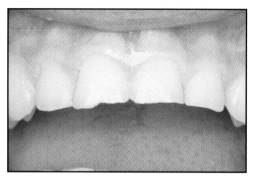

Fig. 3 Chipping of the incisal edges

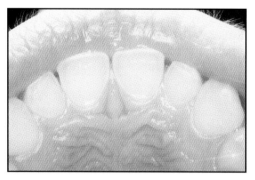

Fig. 4 Areas where the enamel is absent

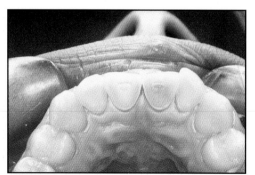

Fig. 5 Exposure of the dental pulp of the maxillary left central incisor

Establishing the diagnosis

History

The need to take an adequate dietary history to explore the extent, frequency and timing of acid consumption has been outlined. A medical history to establish the role, if any, of intrinsic acid is imperative. Children and adolescents with eating disorders are known to be selective with the facts. Dietary enquiries may need to be made on a number of occasions in order to match the history with the dental findings.

The presenting complaint of the child or teenager is of equal importance. This is usually one of the following:
- Sensitivity from the teeth
- Pain from the teeth
- Chipping of the incisal edges
- Fracture of the teeth
- Incisal greying
- Darkening of the teeth.

Examination

Clinical examination of the anterior teeth may reveal any one or all of the following:
- A loss of surface anatomy (fig. 1)
- Increased incisal translucency (fig. 2)
- Chipping of the incisal edges (fig. 3)
- Areas where the enamel is absent (fig. 4)
- Exposure of the pulp (fig. 5).

At the back of the mouth erosion causes a similar loss of surface anatomy, classically with cuspal cupping (fig. 6), and a darkening of the colour of the teeth. However, due to the shape of the teeth, chipping is less frequent. Exposure of the pulp in the posterior teeth of the permanent dentition as a consequence of erosion is almost unheard of whereas pulpal exposure of deciduous molars in cases of severe erosion is seen more frequently (fig. 7).

Management

Once a diagnosis of erosion has been made, management of the condition primarily aims to prevent acid reaching the teeth. If the acid is dietary in origin, advice must centre on altering the diet to remove the cause. Additional recommendations, such as confining the intake of acidic foodstuffs and beverages to mealtimes and never drinking a fruit drink prior to bedtime, need to be given with caution. Monitoring may determine whether the dietary advice has been heeded. However, estimating the progress of wear remains one of the most difficult challenges faced by practitioners today. Despite photographs, study casts and indices, ongoing erosion remains difficult to detect and impossible to quantify. For the permanent dentition the approach of not providing treatment until one is certain erosion has ceased is not realistic. More specifically in today's culture where fruit drinks and carbonated beverages are so readily available many children and adolescents do not and cannot comply with the dietary advice given.

Active restorative intervention is necessary:
- Where there are significant areas of exposed dentine (fig. 8)
- Where there is a risk of tooth fracture (fig. 9)
- If there is hypersensitivity which cannot be controlled by any other means (fig. 10).

The aims of such treatment will be:
- To protect the remaining tooth structure
- Control symptoms and
- To stabilise the occlusion.

A number of materials is available to assist in achieving these aims which differ according to whether deciduous or permanent teeth are being restored.

The deciduous dentition

Treatment of erosion in the deciduous dentition is limited by patient compliance, inadequate enamel and insufficient coronal tissue to provide successful adhesive restorations. In theory it is possible to build up worn deciduous incisors with composite resin, in practice this is rarely done. Provided the worn teeth remain symptom free, they are left unrestored until they are exfoliated (fig. 11). If symptoms arise these teeth are usually removed.

Worn deciduous molars which are sensitive are often not amenable to successful treatment with intra-coronal restorations due to the widespread shallow nature of the erosive lesions (fig. 12). Adhesive materials undoubtedly have more to offer than amalgam in such clinical circumstances and may be successfully used for minimal lesions. However placement of stainless-steel crowns on deciduous molars is frequently the only satisfactory way of providing relief of symptoms, cessation of continued wear and assurance that a tooth may remain *in-situ* until exfoliation.

The permanent dentition

Other articles in this series assess materials currently available to treat wear in the permanent dentition. This remains an area of contention as each clinician tends to favour a particular method. To ensure placement of a satisfactory restoration in the young patient a number of factors need to be borne in mind:
- Enamel loss is characteristically over a wide area of limited thickness (fig. 13)
- Anterior restorations in the mouth of an adolescent are vulnerable to loss, for example contact sports and orthodontic appliances may affect their longevity.

Anterior restorations

Where enamel loss is limited to the incisal aspect of a crown or conversely enamel loss extensive (figs 14, 15), composite resin is the material of choice. This material performs best when placed in bulk and provides an excellent aesthetic

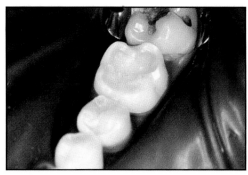

Fig. 6 Wear of a mandibular first molar with loss of surface anatomy

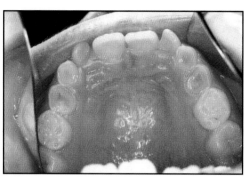

Fig. 7 Pulpal exposure of the maxillary deciduous molars

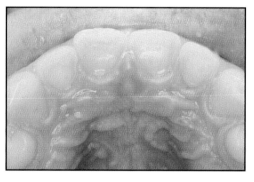

Fig. 8 Significant areas of exposed dentine on the palatal surfaces of the maxillary central incisors

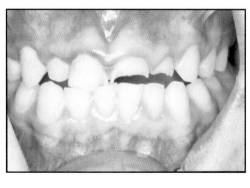

Fig. 9 Fracture of the incisal edges

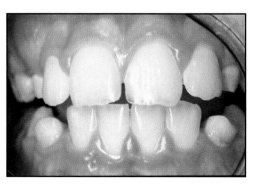

Fig. 10 Widespread loss of enamel leading to hypersensitivity

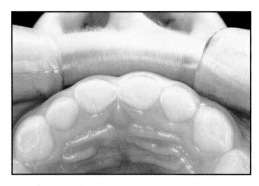

Fig. 11 Worn deciduous incisors

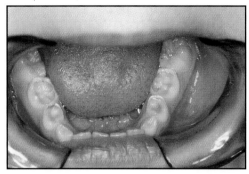

Fig. 12 Worn deciduous molars

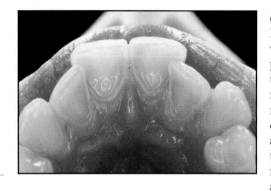

Fig. 13 Enamel lost over a widespread area but of limited thickness

chrome veneers are highly successful (fig. 16): in a series of over three hundred placed by the author in the Paediatric Dental Department at the Eastman Dental Hospital over the past decade, only two veneers have debonded. This reflects the reliability and high bond strengths obtained when using surface-active composite luting agents in conjunction with sand-blasted nickel-chromium alloy. When using opaque versions of these cements, theoretical objections to nickel-chromium alloys on grounds of poor aesthetics are minimal. The preference is for a material which in a number of clinical circumstances, such as resin-retained bridges, has demonstrated its superiority. The clinical procedure is conservative of tooth structure as no preparation is required and cementation is carried out under rubber dam to ensure moisture control. For those operators familiar with the clinical procedure for the cementation of resin-retained bridges, the transference of their skills to cement what, in effect, are multiple individual retainers is straightforward.

A similar method is employed to restore the occlusal surfaces of worn molar teeth (fig. 17). Here a nickel chrome onlay is cemented to the worn occlusal surface of a tooth. Again no tooth preparation is carried out. In the young patient the use of this method is ideal as it conserves the maximum amount of tooth structure with minimal restorative intervention. If at a later date the individual wishes placement of a more aesthetic restoration, a return to how the dentition looked pre-treatment is relatively straightforward. The provision of the nickel-chrome adhesive onlay causing deliberate axial tooth movement has re-created the space lost occlusally through wear.[8]

Tooth surface loss in the younger patient is due primarily to acid erosion. The most significant aetiological factor appears to be the consumption of acidic beverages. Current data indicate that tooth surface loss is widespread in younger patients. The characteristics of the patterns of wear have been described. Young patients often find difficulty in complying with the dietary control necessary to minimise further tooth surface loss.

The restorative principles are conservative relying on adhesive techniques. The durability and predictability of adhesive nickel-chromium

result. In individuals where the pattern of enamel loss is more classical in its distribution involving the palatal surfaces of upper anterior teeth, composite resin is difficult to apply, demanding to finish and liable to fracture. The claim that easy repair makes composite an ideal material for use in this situation is countered by the almost certain need for frequent repairs and regular maintenance.

Frequently it is necessary to restore the incisal aspect of an upper anterior tooth with composite resin and employ a more durable, stronger material to restore the palatal surfaces. The two materials most suitable for this purpose are yellow gold and nickel-chromium alloys. Nickel-

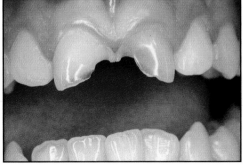

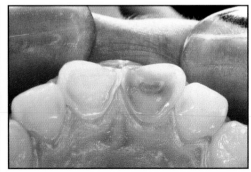

Figs. 14 and 15 The labial and palatal views of two extensively worn maxillary central incisors

1 Black G V. *A work on operative dentistry in two volumes.* Chicago. Medico-dental publishing company, 1908.

2 O'Brien M. *Children's Dental Health in the United Kingdom, 1993.* London: OPCS HMSO.

3 British Soft Drinks Association. *Report of Seminar in Heidelberg, 1991; Factsheet number 9-7.91.*

4 Rugg-Gunn A J, Lennon M A, Brown J. Sugar consumption in the United Kingdom. *Br Dent J* 1986; **161**: 359-364.

5 Shaw L. Personal communication, 1998.

6 Millward A, Shaw I, Smith A J, Rippin J W, Harrington E. The distribution and severity of tooth wear and the relationship between erosion and dietary constituents in a group of children. *Int J Paed Dent* 1994; **4**: 151-157.

7 O'Sullivan E A, Curzon M E J, Roberts G J, Milla P J, Stringer M D. Gastroesophageal reflux in children and its relationship to erosion of primary and permanent teeth. *Eur J Oral Sci* 1998; **106**: 765-769.

8 Harley K E, Ibbetson R J. Dental anomalies — are adhesive castings the solution? *Br Dent J* 1993; **174**: 15-22.

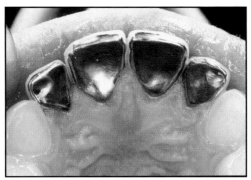

Fig. 16 Nickel-chromium veneers on the palatal surfaces of the maxillary incisors

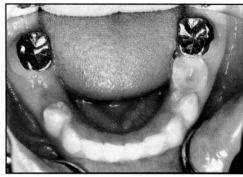

Fig. 17 Nickel-chromium onlays placed on the mandibular first molars

veneers make them the method of choice where teeth require protection against further damage. When the incisal edges of the maxillary incisors have been lost, composite resin is effective only when used in sufficient bulk. The restorative management parallels that for adults with adhesive techniques being used whenever possible.

The final parts of this series will discuss the principles of treatment planning for the restorative care of those affected by tooth surface loss. The next article describes how treatment can be ordered to deliver it effectively and the strategies that may be used to create interocclusal space when clinical crown height is lacking.

9 Treatment planning

R. Ibbetson

An effective treatment plan is dependent on gathering information from the history, examination and special tests, such as radiographs and vitality testing, and analysing it to make a diagnosis. In restorative dentistry diagnoses are frequently multiple: successful treatment planning depends on accurate diagnoses and appropriate decision-making. The series has emphasised the importance of effective prevention, it has also recognised that restoration may be needed to protect the remaining tooth structure.

The treatment plan

The treatment plan should take the patient and dentist to the point where disease is controlled and the dentition functional and stable. Absolute stability is not achievable: all restorative work deteriorates to the point where failure becomes inevitable. Restorative work cannot be guaranteed for a patient's lifetime and no outrageous claims for longevity should be made.

The dentist must be aware of the patient's wishes. Frequently they ask the dentist to select the treatment. Rather they should be encouraged to make decisions for themselves while the dentist's role is to provide the information. Very often the patient's expectations of treatment are different from our own.[1,2]

In the worn dentition, it may be difficult to determine the major aetiological factor. Commonly, more than one type of wear is present. It is rare to find a patient with tooth surface loss without at least some element being caused by acid erosion.[3] Management of the patient whose teeth are worn poses the following questions:

1. Does the patient perceive that there is a problem?
2. Is the wear currently active: if so, is it rapid or slow?
3. Will the patient cooperate in a preventive approach to management? If so, how easy will it be to monitor its success?
4. Is the wear so severe that restoration is required?
5. If restoration is required, is there sufficient crown height and do occlusal relationships allow reasonable form and stability to be achieved?
6. Are other teeth likely to require restoration in the short to middle term?

The answers determine the strategy for management. They all require decisions and patient involvement, particularly with regard to their possible long-term consequences as was discussed in Part 7 on failures.

The first stage in developing a treatment plan is to decide which teeth have a hopelessly poor prognosis, which are sound with a good prognosis and finally which teeth require treatment and why. This may not always be evident immediately as some teeth may require investigation to make or confirm a diagnosis, while decisions regarding periodontally compromised teeth may be influenced by the patient's efforts in plaque control.

Treatment plan -v- sequence of treatment

Once the treatment plan, the ultimate goal, is known, the dentist must establish a course that will reach it, *the sequence of treatment.*

Treatment plans should be written down for both dentists' and patients' benefit and the dentist should commit the sequence of treatment to paper. This may show illogicalities: if these are not identified treatment may become unduly complicated or impossible to deliver. For example, it is wise to complete placement of any necessary amalgam restorations before providing the patient with an occlusal splint because re-fitting an existing splint over a newly placed restoration is a complication that is better avoided.

Sequence of treatment

The treatment can be broken down into a sequence of stages. These are:

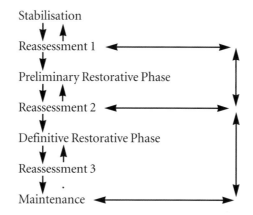

Stabilisation
Reassessment 1
Preliminary Restorative Phase
Reassessment 2
Definitive Restorative Phase
Reassessment 3
Maintenance

The need for re-assessment

During treatment the effects of what has been done should be periodically reviewed. This allows either the dentist or patient to retire

> **Restorative dental care is planned in a series of stages. Casts mounted in an articulator are used as an essential part of this process.**

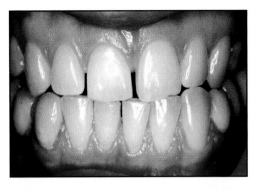

Fig. 1 Labial view of anterior teeth showing chipping of incisal edges of maxillary incisors

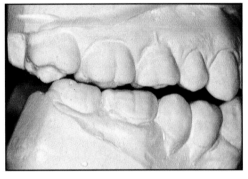

Fig. 2 Incisal edges of maxillary anterior teeth demonstrating acid erosion

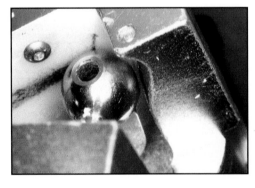

Fig. 3 Mounted casts showing initial contact in the retruded axis position

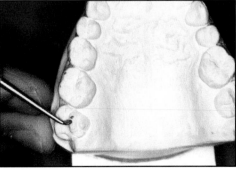

Fig. 4 The 'condyle' has moved away from the rear wall of the condylar housing by 'translation' as the casts have slid into ICP

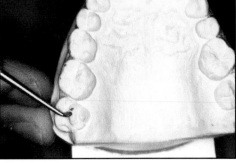

Fig. 5 Trial adjustment of the casts to eliminate the slide between retruded and intercuspal

honourably from active treatment if that seems appropriate. For example, the patient's plaque control may not reach an appropriate standard. This is clearly important in its own right but is also a useful barometer of a patient's level of interest and commitment. Efficacy of plaque control should be measured by bleeding scores not by plaque scores. Plaque scores inform only about performance on the day while bleeding scores give a longer term view.

Sometimes it becomes apparent that the patient may not wish to continue with treatment or the need for the planned work has diminished. Organisation of treatment into stages allows convenient points to be reached when the dentition is relatively stable. If the dentist or patient agree, the patient can enter a maintenance programme and be reviewed periodically. The other phases of treatment are organised to allow a logical progression toward completion of the treatment plan.

Stabilisation phase

The aims are the resolution of any acute problems and the stabilisation or elimination of active disease. Included are:

- Relieving pain and discomfort.
- Instituting effective plaque control procedures: this may include some initial non-surgical periodontal treatment.
- Eliminating active carious lesions.
- Extracting teeth that have a hopeless prognosis.
- Any necessary gross occlusal adjustment, for example a grossly over-erupted tooth.
- Replacement of missing teeth. This may be needed because of appearance or because few posterior teeth are in occlusion preventing there being a sufficiently stable position of closure. If teeth are replaced early in treatment, the prosthesis should generally be provisional with the definitive one being provided during the final restorative phase.

It is prudent to avoid being fully committed to extensive treatment of a patient too soon. Generally existing crown and bridgework should not be removed early in treatment. Dentists often do this on grounds of its being ill-fitting and wishing to provide better temporary restorations: most temporary coverage does not achieve this aim. Once existing work has been removed there is a commitment to complete treatment which a lack of patient compliance can make difficult.

Re-assessment 1

This is a review of whether the patient's condition has stabilised. Is the patient comfortable, are they are able to accept treatment, what improvement has been made in their standard of plaque control? Does the patient appear to be interested in treatment? It may be that a lack of response or difficulties in accepting treatment require revision of the long-term goals.

Preliminary restorative phase

Treatment is directed toward:

- Investigating individual teeth, providing cores and new plastic restorations as necessary.
- Any definitive endodontic treatment.
- Non-surgical periodontal therapy.
- A full analysis of the occlusion.

The clinical examination of the occlusion is supplemented by an extra-oral analysis using accurate study casts made from alginate impressions and a facebow transfer so that the maxillary cast can be mounted in an articulator. An inter-occlusal record taken in the retruded axis position (RAP) is needed to relate the mandibular cast to the maxillary and thereby to the hinge axis of the articulator. The casts are used to assess in more detail the extent of the tooth surface loss and to determine which teeth might benefit from further restoration. Consideration then must be given to determining exactly what difficulties may complicate the proposed restorations.

Re-assessment 2

A further review of progress is made and any concerns that the dentist or patient has over the final phase of treatment can be discussed.

There are a number of aspects to re-assess:

- Disease control
- The aims of the definitive restorative phase
- The position of the teeth
- The crown height available
- The position of mandibular closure and the jaw relationships.

Periodontal condition and disease control

There should be no active disease. Homecare should be commensurate with supporting the final restorative phase of treatment. If there are specific sites of periodontal concern remaining despite good plaque control, there may be indications for periodontal surgery. However, the traditional goal of pocket elimination by surgical means is becoming increasingly hard to substantiate.

The definitive restorative phase

The aims of the final restorative stage should be well defined. Decisions about whether to provide indirect restorations for patients with worn teeth are based on:

- Aesthetics
- Occlusal stability
- Protection of the remaining tooth structure.

Two sets of study casts should be available that are mounted accurately in the articulator. One acts as a baseline record. The second is available for rehearsing treatment, for example crown lengthening surgery, occlusal adjustment or diagnostic waxing.

The position of the teeth

Assessment of the casts or a diagnostic wax-up may show that one or more teeth are malposi-

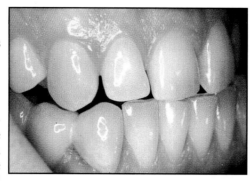

Fig. 6 Intercuspal position prior to occlusal adjustment

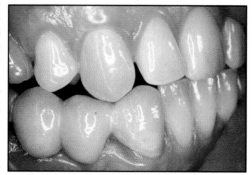

Fig. 7 Intercuspal position following elimination of the slide from retruded to intercuspal showing a small increase in overjet

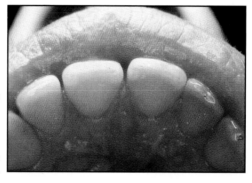

Fig. 8 Incisal edges of the maxillary incisors restored with adhesive composite restorations

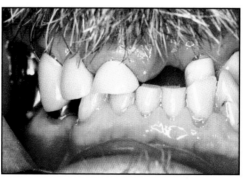

Fig. 9 Patient with worn and restored anterior teeth, missing teeth and an uneven occlusal plane. The teeth are in their intercuspal position

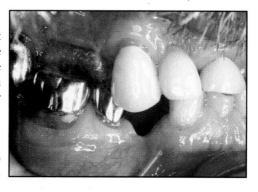

Fig. 10 Buccal view of the teeth in occlusion

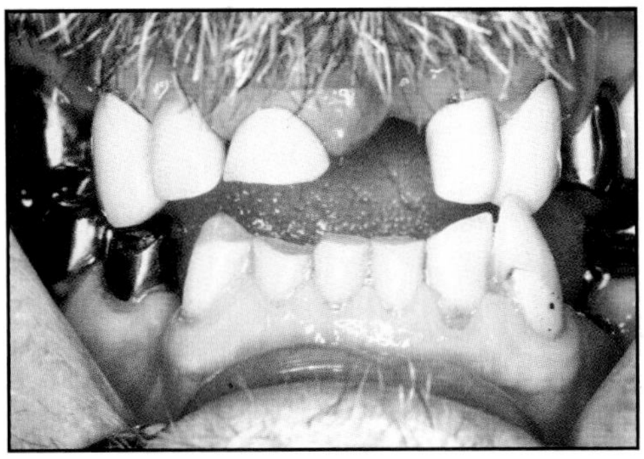

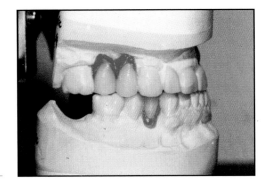

Fig. 11 The mandibular relation in the retruded contact position

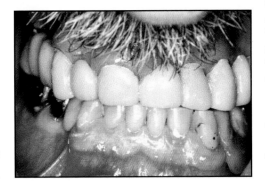

Fig. 12 A diagnostic wax-up and set-up in RAP at an increased occlusal vertical dimension

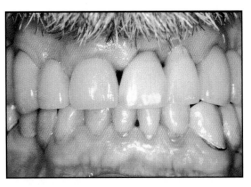

Fig. 13 A labial view of the maxillary provisional prosthesis made from a matrix of the diagnostic wax-up

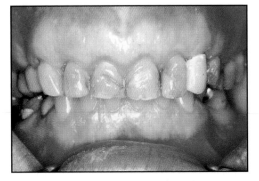

Fig. 14 An anterior view of the final anterior restorations

Fig. 15 A middle-aged patient with a dentition affected by tooth surface loss

tioned and sometimes orthodontics can be helpful. Orthodontics in the pre-restorative management of the worn dentition is discussed in Part 10 of the series. It needs to be planned jointly by the restorative dentist and the orthodontist. It must be established whether permanent retention will be necessary post-treatment: it is frequently required after teeth have been moved in adult patients.

Crown height
The study casts and the wax-up provide a very good idea of clinical crown height. If the teeth are too short, aesthetics, retention and resistance form and occlusal stability are all likely to be compromised. A surgical crown lengthening procedure should be considered to increase the height available. This aspect of treatment will be described in Part 11. Where teeth have large cores, it is important that the margins of the final crowns are placed apical to the margins of the cores on sound dentine — 2 mm is considered sufficient.[4] Frequently this is impossible without prior crown lengthening.

Creating space for restoring worn teeth by control of the jaw relationship
There are a number of other ways of creating space to allow restoration of short teeth. These are by:
- Altering the position of mandibular closure while maintaining the existing vertical dimension of occlusion
- Increasing the vertical dimension of occlusion
- Reversing the changes that have taken place in the position of the teeth as a result of the wear through relative axial tooth movement.

Sometimes a combination of more than one of these approaches is necessary. In all instances, it is important to determine a stable RAP before planning the definitive restorations. This requires a period of wear of an occlusal splint. The details of this appliance can be found in Part 3 of this series.

Alteration of the position of mandibular closure
This is considered when there is need to restore teeth in the anterior part of the mouth and the rest of the dentition is generally sound. The change in the position of mandibular closure is effected by occlusal adjustment. The aim is to create a new intercuspal position (ICP) some way distal to but at the same vertical dimension as the existing one. The feasibility of doing this depends on the nature of the discrepancy between RAP and ICP: there must be significant mandibular translation between the two positions for it to be a possibility.

The magnitude of this type of movement is hard to determine from intra-oral examination. It is seen best on mounted study casts by determining the change in the position of the articulator 'condyles' relative to their condylar housings when the casts are slid into the intercuspal position from the retruded axis position. The only reliable way of determining whether elimination of the anterior slide would create space anteriorly is by rehearsing it on the second set of mounted casts.

Figures 1 to 8 show a 30-year-old female who had begun to wear the incisal edges of her maxillary central incisors primarily through dietary erosion such that the incisal edges had begun to chip. Figure 1 shows the edge-to-edge incisal relationship in ICP. The mandibular incisors occluded against the worn incisal edges. There was no space available to allow the restoration and protection of these maxillary teeth. The patient was found to have a significant horizontal component to the slide from retruded into intercuspal (figs 3, 4, 6, 7). Adjustment of the posterior teeth to eliminate the discrepancy produced a new intercuspal position with the mandible positioned further distally increasing the overjet sufficiently to allow conservative restoration of the incisal edges of the maxillary incisors with composite resin (fig. 8).

Increasing the vertical dimension of occlusion

This is the traditional way of creating space for the restoration of worn teeth. The decision to increase the vertical dimension of occlusion brings with it the obligation to restore a large number of teeth to ensure that the teeth in both arches have antagonists on mandibular closure. Treatment is demanding for both operator and patient with many hours being spent by the patient in the dental chair: it is only undertaken when simpler alternatives are inappropriate.

Increasing the vertical dimension not only provides space for restorations but also gives scope for levelling a disordered occlusal plane. Figures 9 to 15 show a middle-aged man in whom increasing the vertical dimension of occlusion created space for restorations while at the same time producing a level occlusal plane.

Total face height measured in the rest position has traditionally been thought of as relatively constant. However, this is not the case. If mandibular rest position were thought of as being consistent with minimal jaw muscle activity, electromyographic studies carried out in the early 1960s by Ramfjord indicated that low levels of muscle activity were found over a range of about a centimetre in most people.[5] Clinical experience has indicated that moderate increases in the vertical dimension of occlusion are well tolerated by patients as long as they are accompanied by a stable position of mandibular closure together with anterior guidance that provides separation of the posterior teeth on mandibular movement.[6] This view is supported by what little research is available.[7]

Aesthetic limitations on lengthening the teeth incisally often make an adjunctive surgical

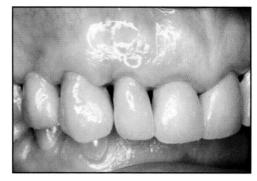

Fig. 16 The same patient following surgical crown lengthening and placement of metal-ceramic crowns. The wide embrasures are evident

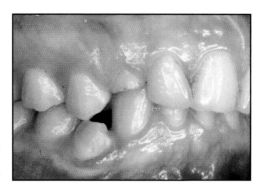

Fig. 17 Buccal view of patient with worn deciduous canine

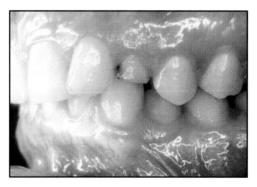

Fig. 18 Buccal view of patient with worn deciduous canine

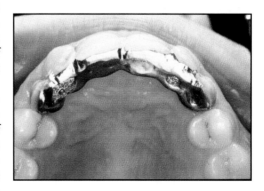

Fig. 19 Palatal view of cemented 'Dahl' appliance on c321/12c

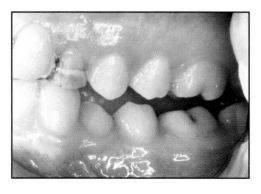

Fig. 20 Buccal view of patient occluding on anterior appliance

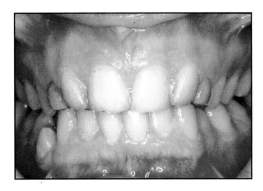

Fig 21 Following axial tooth movement, posterior occlusion re-established

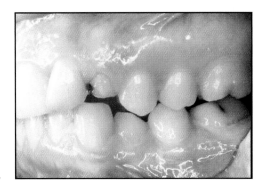

Fig. 22 Following removal of the appliance showing the space available to allow restoration

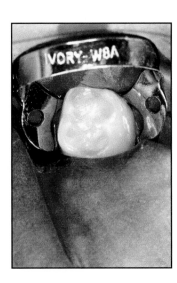

Fig. 23 Tooth surface loss having affected the occlusal surface of a mandibular molar in a 17 year-old

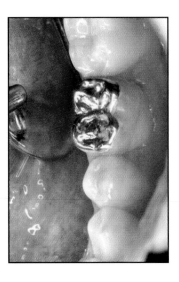

Fig. 24 Mandibular first molar restored with adhesive metal casting cemented at an increased vertical dimension of occlusion

crown lengthening procedure necessary if the appearance is to be reasonable (fig. 15). The potential aesthetic disadvantages are that in moving the gingival margin apically, it comes to rest on a narrower portion of the root. This makes the embrasure spaces larger which may be difficult to disguise using the final restorations and so-called 'black-hole' disease may result (fig. 16).

Deliberate axial tooth movement

The method was originally described by Dahl.[8] He used removable bite-planes to intrude worn anterior teeth that he wished to crown without having to restore the posterior dentition. His original description was of treating individuals in their sixties. However in the past 20 years, it has been applied to patients of all ages affected by tooth wear. Developments, particularly the use of tooth-borne appliances luted to the teeth using glass ionomer cement, has led to increased predictability and patient compliance. Such an appliance is shown in the treatment of someone whose retained deciduous maxillary canines had become very worn and the opposing canines over-erupted (figs 18 to 23).

Casts mounted in an articulator prior to treatment are used to assess where the teeth will be after axial movement. It is important that there are stable occlusal contacts after treatment otherwise the teeth will re-erupt.

The technique is often used to simplify the full reconstruction of the worn dentition. An appliance cemented to the maxillary anterior teeth creates space posteriorly allowing easy access for the placement of any necessary cores. Once the axial tooth movement is complete and the posterior teeth have re-established contact, sufficient space will have been created anteriorly to allow these teeth to be restored. This is followed by the placement of the necessary posterior crowns. This approach will be described more fully in Part 12 of the series.

Relative axial tooth movement, reversing the changes that accompany wear, allows simpler restorative procedures. Figures 24 and 25 show the occlusal surface of a lower first molar tooth in a late teenager. The tooth had been eroded by carbonated drink and there was no clearance on closure between it and its antagonist. The tooth was restored with an adhesive nickel-chrome occlusal casting. This was around 1.5 mm thick and after cementation was initially the only site of occlusal contact. Two weeks later, axial tooth movement had taken place and all the teeth had intercuspal contacts.

The final restorations

The aims are to provide optimal aesthetics, reasonable function and ensure that any restorations placed are compatible with the patient maintaining themselves in a disease-free state. The previous investigative stages will, in con-

1 Brisman A S. Esthetics: a comparison of dentists' and patients' concepts. *J Am Dent Assoc* 1980; **100**: 345-352.

2 Neumann L M, Christensen C, Cavanaugh C. Dental esthetic satisfaction in adults. *J Am Dent Assoc* 1989; **118**: 565 -570.

3 Smith B G N. Some facets of tooth wear. *Ann R Aust Coll Dent Surg* 1991; **11**: 37-51.

4 Hoag E P, Dwyer T G. A comparative evaluation of three post and core techniques. *J Prosthet Dent* 1982; **47**: 177-181.

5 Garnick J J, Ramfjord S P. Rest position. *J Prosthet Dent* 1962; **12**: 895-911.

6 Ibbetson R J, Setchell D J. Treatment of the worn dentition 2. *Dent Update* 1989; **17**: 300-307.

7 Rivera-Morales W C, Mohl N D. Relationship of occlusal vertical dimension to the health of the masticatory system. *J Prosthet Dent* 1991; **65**: 547-553.

8 Dahl B L, Krogstad O, Karlsen K. An alternative treatment in cases with advanced localised attrition. *J Oral Rehab* 1975: **2**: 209-214.

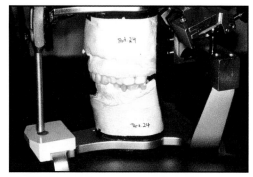

Fig. 25 Diagnostic wax-up made at the beginning of the definitive restorative stage

junction with the patient's wishes, have determined which teeth would benefit from restoration. Diagnostic waxing forms an essential part of the planning.

Diagnostic waxing

Restorative treatment is much more predictable when the outcome can be envisaged (fig. 25). It is also gives the patient an idea of the final result and encourages realistic expectations. Specifically diagnostic waxing will:

- Allow dentist and patient to see a mock-up of the final restorations.
- Indicate if there is sufficient crown height to give adequate retention and resistance form in the preparations, reasonable aesthetics and adequate occlusal form.
- Show where occlusal plane discrepancies (for example, slightly over-erupted antagonist teeth) need correction if a desirable occlusal scheme is to be achieved and optimal aesthetics produced.

The wax-up provides a number of additional advantages. It can guide tooth preparation using it to make matrices that are either used to evaluate the preparations or as templates for the temporary coverage. The temporaries have ostensibly the same form as the final restorations so they can be used to check the appropriateness of the tooth reduction by measuring their thickness. The temporary crowns can also be used to rehearse the final result. It is an interesting thought that dentists are trained as undergraduates to make a wax 'try-in' for a removable prosthesis. However it seems this is rarely advised for a fixed prosthesis or a number of crowns. The temporary restorations fulfil that role and the final crowns should present few surprises either to the dentist or the patient.

Re-assessment 3

This final review is an evaluation of whether the original aims of treatment have been met and whether further active restorative care is required. If all is satisfactory, the patient enters the maintenance phase. The details of which were described in Part 6 of the series.

This article has described the importance of determining, in conjunction with the patient their restorative needs and has outlined an approach to the delivery of care. The way in which teeth wear, together with their inherent eruptive potential, can combine to create particular difficulties in restoration. They often present broad, flat functional surfaces where their relationships with antagonists make it difficult to create adequate space for effective restoration. Various strategies that can be used to create space for restorative purposes have been outlined. The benefits of deliberate axial tooth movement as a conservative method for management have been described. Orthodontics and surgical crown lengthening can also be valuable adjuncts to restorative care. The next two articles in the series will discuss in more detail their use and limitations in the restorative management of worn teeth.

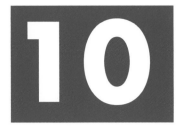

Orthodontic options

R. D. Evans[1]

Previous articles in this series have described the changes that take place when teeth wear. If this is caused by attrition, slowly progressive erosion or a combination of both, there is invariably compensation by tooth eruption and dentoalveolar growth to maintain occlusal contact in maximum intercuspation.[1,2] When the tooth wear primarily affects the palatal surfaces of the maxillary incisors and less frequently the lower incisal edges, contact is maintained in maximum intercuspation. This, unfortunately, means that often there will be insufficient interocclusal space to place restorations if these are needed. This can be created in a number of ways:

• Tooth preparation with the consequent removal of more tooth tissue
• Changing the jaw relationship
• Conventional orthodontic treatment using combinations of fixed and/or removable appliances
• Fixed or removable bite platforms – originally described by Dahl.[3]

The possibility of orthodontic treatment is often not considered for adults. This is either on grounds of potential difficulties in treatment or the acceptability of appliances to adult patients, particularly those that are fixed. However, orthodontic treatment is increasingly common in older age groups. Optimal aesthetic results are achieved when teeth are correctly positioned. Restorative procedures can be facilitated by orthodontics: for example, the re-creation of the space that would have been occupied by maxillary lateral incisors in patients affected by hypodontia.

The previous article discussed ways in which space could be created when worn teeth need restoration. One approach centred on changing the jaw relationship and consequently the position of mandibular closure. The second described the application of Dahl's work which uses bite platforms or modifications of them to produce relative axial tooth movement: this is essentially a type of orthodontic treatment. Conventional orthodontic treatment may also be useful in the prerestorative treatment of worn teeth allowing the relationship between them to be altered so that restoration becomes easier or sometimes possible when previously it was not.

Some of the changes which occur in the relationships of worn teeth can be corrected by orthodontic treatment. This can improve the quality of restorative care.

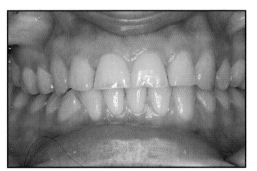

Fig 1a Labial view of teeth worn through a combination of erosion and attrition

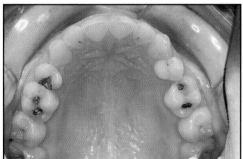

Fig1b Palatal view of the worn maxillary anterior teeth

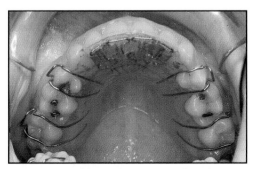

Fig 1c Removable appliance to procline the maxillary incisors

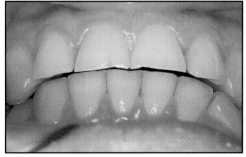

Fig 1d The increased overjet produced by the orthodontic treatment

[1]Consultant Orthodontist, Eastman Dental Hospital, University College London Hospitals Trust and The Hospital for Sick Children, Great Ormond Street & Honorary Senior Lecturer, Eastman Dental Institute for Oral Health Care Sciences, University of London, 256 Gray's Inn Road, London WC1X 8LD

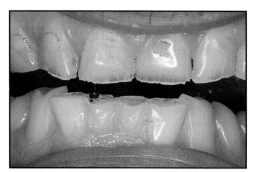

Fig 2a Labial view of dentition affected by erosion caused by bulimia

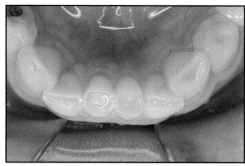

Fig 2b The worn incisal edges of the mandibular anterior teeth

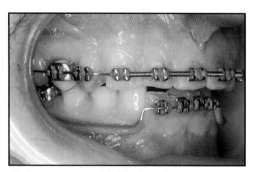

Fig 2c Treatment with fixed appliances

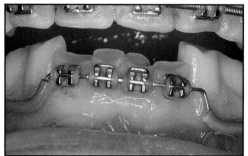

Fig 2d Labial view to show lower incisor intrusion to allow restoration

The orthodontic approach

Before embarking on treatment it is essential that the case is considered by both orthodontic and restorative specialists to clearly identify the aims and often more importantly, the limitations of treatment.[4,5] A number of orthodontic techniques is available to create localised interocclusal space and the decision about which is the most appropriate will depend on a careful examination of the accompanying malocclusion. In cases of localised anterior tooth wear, interocclusal space can be created by careful overbite reduction and in certain cases lower incisor retraction. The tooth movements required to reduce an overbite[6] include:

- Upper and lower incisor and canine intrusion
- Upper and lower incisor proclination
- Premolar and molar extrusion.

If orthodontic treatment is being carried out to correct other features of the malocclusion such as crowding, spacing and overjet reduction, the creation of anterior interocclusal space forms a part of the overall treatment. In this situation the way in which the overbite is reduced will depend on a number of factors including the determinants of the malocclusion and the age of the patient. In children, where there is remaining growth, it is common to extrude the premolars and molars as a way of reducing the overbite. The increase in the lower face height and backward rotation of the mandible is compensated by continued facial growth. In adult patients, premolars and molars should not be extruded as the result can be potentially unsta-

ble in the absence of significant remaining facial growth. In contrast, the orthodontic treatment should be focused, in general, on incisor and canine intrusion.

When the aim of the orthodontic treatment is purely to create anterior interocclusal space the techniques previously described can be adapted to the individual case. A combination of upper incisor proclination, lower incisor intrusion and in certain cases lower incisor retraction is effective. This can allow restorations to be placed on the palatal surfaces of the upper incisors and lower incisal edges. These must provide contacts on mandibular closure to ensure stability of the teeth in their new positions.

The choice of removable, fixed appliances or a combination of both will depend on the type of tooth movements required. Springs incorporated into removable appliances are only capable of producing tipping movements. If all that is required is upper incisor proclination, a removable appliance with suitable stainless steel springs will produce the desired tooth movements. Fixed appliances allow three-dimensional control permitting intrusion, extrusion, translation (bodily movement) or torqueing (root movement) of the teeth. Intrusion of incisors requires light, precisely directed forces, around 15 grams for a lower incisor and 20 grams for an upper incisor. Excessive force may result in apical root resorption and root shortening. The choice between 'full arch' or 'segmental' mechanics will depend on the primary determinants of the overbite and desired tooth movements and can be adapted to the individual case. A recent study has shown that neither technique is particularly associated with apical root resorption.[7] However, the use of fixed appliances to reduce the overbite is complicated and requires expertise in fixed appliance technique.

These principles are illustrated in the following three cases:

Case 1 (Figs 1a–d). An upper removable appliance has been used to procline the upper incisors. If the incisors are initially well aligned, space will develop between the teeth. This may or may not need restorative intervention. In this particular case the base-plate of the upper appliance was adjusted to provide even contact with the lower incisal edges to prevent an increase in the overbite.

Case 2 (Figs 2a–d). In this case of bulimia affecting a 45 year old man, the upper incisors have been proclined and the lower incisors intruded with fixed appliances.

Case 3 (Figs 3a–d). To create anterior interocclusal space to restore 21|12 in the presence of a Class III incisor relationship, the lower incisors have been retracted following the extraction of one lower incisor.

Some adjustment to the individual tooth positions may be required to equalise the interocclusal space. This is achieved by placing detailing bends in the archwire to produce the ideal final tooth positions.

Having created adequate interocclusal space it is important to maintain it until either the provisional or definitive restorations are placed. It is possible to restore the damaged surfaces of teeth with the fixed appliances in place — the appliances can be removed after the restorations are in place.

One single technique is not suitable for all situations. It is important to consider the aetiology of the increased overbite and age of the patient before deciding on the most appropriate treatment. For many patients where the only problem is anterior tooth wear it may not be acceptable to wear either removable or fixed appliances, especially for periods of up to 12 months, although the patient should be allowed to make that decision for themselves.

The 'Dahl' approach

An alternative method of creating an anterior interocclusal space involves the use of fixed anterior bite raising appliances: this was originally described by Dahl. This technique involves placing an anterior bite raising appliance or bite platform which has been shown in an implant-cephalometric study[8] to result in intrusion of the anterior teeth by an average of 1.05 mm, and extrusion or eruption of the remaining teeth, averaging 1.47 mm after 6–14 months, without causing undue incisor proclination.[9] It was shown that the increase in occlusal face height was variable, averaging 1.9 mm with the post treatment decrease confined to a 6-month period.[10] This type of appliance differs from a conventional flat anterior bite plane built into an upper removable appliance in that the anterior and posterior parts of

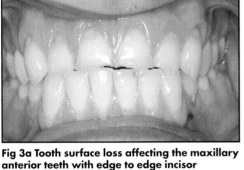

Fig 3a Tooth surface loss affecting the maxillary anterior teeth with edge to edge incisor relationship

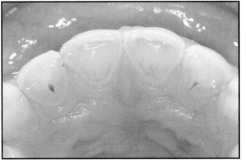

Fig 3b Maxillary anterior teeth showing tooth surface loss caused by acid erosion

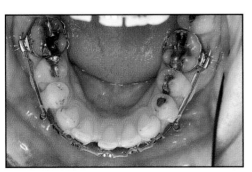

Fig 3c Mandibular fixed appliance in place

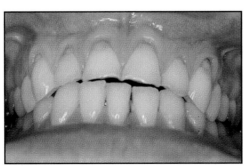

Fig 3d Retraction and intrusion of the lower labial segment creating space for restoration of the maxillary anterior teeth

1 Berry D C, Poole D F G. Attrition: possible mechanisms of compensation. *J Oral Rehabil* 1976; 3: 201-206.

2 Crothers A, Sandham A. Vertical height differences in subjects with severe dental wear. *Eur J Orthod* 1993; 15: 519-525.

3 Dahl B L, Krogstad O, Karlsen K. An alternative treatment in cases with advanced localised attrition. *J Oral Rehab* 1975; 2: 209-214.

4 Beckett H A, Evans R D. The interface between orthodontics and restorative dentistry in the management of anterior tooth surface loss. *Br J Orthodont* 1994; 21: 231-237.

5 Evans R D. Orthodontics and the creation of localised interocclusal space in cases of anterior tooth wear. *Eur J Prosthdont Rest Dent* 1997; 5: 169-173.

6 Bennett J C, McLaughlin R P. Management of deep overbite with a preadjusted edgewise system. *J Clin Orthodont* 1990; 24: 684-696.

7 Costopolous G, Nanda R. An evaluation of root resorption incident to orthodontic intrusion. *Am J Orthod Dentofacial Orthped* 1996; 105: 543-548.

8 Dahl B L, Krogstad O. The effect of a partial bite-raising splint on the occlusal face height. An x-ray cephalometric study in human adults. *Acta Odontol Scand* 1982; 40: 17-24.

9 Dahl B L, Krogstad O. The effect of a partial bite raising splint on the inclination of the upper and lower front teeth. *Acta Odontol Scand* 1983; 41: 311-314.

10 Dahl B L, Krogstad O. Long-term observations of an increased occlusal face height obtained by a combined orthodontic/prosthetic approach. *J Oral Rehab* 1985; **12**: 171-176.

11 Briggs P, Bishop K, Dejmal S. The clinical evolution of the 'Dahl Principle'. *Br Dent J* 1997; **183**: 171-176.

12 Ricketts N J, Smith B G N. Clinical techniques for producing and monitoring minor axial tooth movement. *Eur J Prosthodont Rest Dent* 1994; **2**: 5-9.

13 Ricketts N J, Smith B G N. Minor axial tooth movement in preparation for fixed prostheses. *Eur J Prosthodont Rest Dent* 1993; **1**: 145-149.

14 Darbar U R, Hemmings K W. Treatment of localised anterior tooth wear with composite restorations at an increased occlusal vertical dimension. *Dent Update* 1997; **24**: 72-75.

15 Ibbetson R J, Setchell D J. Treatment of the worn dentition: 2. *Dent Update* 1989; **16**: 300-307.

the dental arch are able to move independently of each other. The technique continues to evolve with recent reports describing the use of composite resin both directly and indirectly, intermediate fixed metal prostheses, definitive individual adhesive restorations, intermediate temporary full coverage restorations and finally definitive conventional full coverage restorations.[11–15] Unfortunately, to date there are no published long-term studies evaluating the outcome of many of these new approaches. However, these principles have been in use at the Eastman Dental Institute and Hospital for nearly 20 years in the prerestorative treatment of patients affected by tooth surface loss. They have proved predictable, well tolerated by patients and produce few complications.

Conventional orthodontics should be considered as a way of creating localised interocclusal space in cases of anterior tooth wear if there are other aspects of the malocclusion that require treatment. The 'Dahl' approach is very effective at creating interocclusal space but can-

not deal with malaligned teeth. It is therefore important to consider a full orthodontic assessment in cases of anterior tooth wear as it forms an alternative strategy for creating the space necessary for restorations. If appropriate, orthodontic treatment should be offered to patients affected by tooth surface loss as it can reduce the complexities of the restorative procedures.

A theme has been evident in many of the articles in this series that short teeth create restorative difficulties in retention and resistance form, structural durability and may compromise aesthetics. The strategies that have been described for creating space between opposing teeth may, by themselves, not be sufficient to overcome these problems. Surgical crown lengthening may be necessary, involving the dentist working with another specialist in planning restorative work. The next article in the series describes the scope and limitations of surgical crown lengthening in the management of patients with worn teeth.

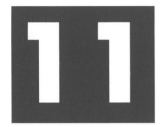

Surgical crown lengthening

V. J. Ward[1]

One of the themes of this series has been the changes that take place in the relationship of the teeth as they wear. This creates many of the difficulties that compromise the form of restorations, their occlusal relationships and adequate retention and resistance form. Part 9 described the strategies that were available for altering the occlusal relationships to provide more space and facilitate the restorative procedures.

Relative axial tooth movement not only creates space but reverses the changes in the position of the teeth that accompany wear. This results in the gingival tissues moving with the tooth so that reasonable clinical crown length often results. However, when it is intended to provide restorative treatment at the existing vertical dimension of occlusion, difficulties in providing adequate interocclusal clearance may so compromise the results that surgical crown lengthening becomes necessary. There are, however, finite limits as to how much lengthening of the clinical crowns of teeth can be achieved by surgical means. A further strategy for creating the necessary interocclusal clearance with adequate crown height is by increasing the vertical dimension of occlusion. However, there are again limits as to how much height and clearance can be gained by this technique. This is not so much related to patient tolerance but rather the adverse effect that it can have on the relationship of the anterior teeth. As the vertical dimension is increased, the mandible rotates so that it comes to lie further distally. This increases the overjet and can be sufficient to make contacts between the anterior teeth and hence adequate occlusal stability and anterior guidance difficult to achieve. The net result of the limitations with both techniques is that they are frequently combined to allow adequate crown height with sufficient interocclusal clearance to be achieved in preparations.

The clinical height of the crown of a tooth can be increased by the removal of the coronal portion of the periodontium together with crestal bone, using standard periodontal flap procedures. It is always necessary to use a flap procedure, unless the clinical crown is shorter than the anatomical crown, in which case gingivectomy procedures will suffice.

When planning how much tissue to remove, there must be at least 3 mm between the most apical extension of any restorative margin and the crest of the alveolar bone. This figure is derived from human autopsy material which showed:[1]

- An average sulcus depth of 0.69 mm
- An average epithelial attachment of 0.97 mm
- An average connective tissue attachment of 1.07 mm.

These proportions between bone crest, epithelium and connective tissue attachment remained constant. The sum of the connective tissue and epithelial attachments ie the distance from the alveolar crest to the base of the gingival sulcus was referred as the 'biological width'.[2] This may vary between individuals but remains constant for one person.

Restorative procedures which encroach upon this always cause resorption of crestal bone and migration of the junction epithelium until the necessary 'biological width' has been re-established. The need to maintain it influences the amount of bone removal required during crown lengthening surgery. Once the clinician has decided on the clinical crown height necessary to restore the tooth, not only must sufficient bone be removed to achieve the desired crown height but the biological width must be taken into account. Failure to do so will result in inflammation. Where gingival tissue is thin, this can lead to recession and exposure of crown margins originally placed within the sulcus with an adverse effect on the aesthetics (fig. 1). Where the gingiva is thick, rather than recession, hyperplasia and chronic inflammation will be the result (fig. 2).

It may not be possible to remove the amount of tissue which is necessary to produce the desired crown height. Anatomical factors may limit bone removal and hence potential crown

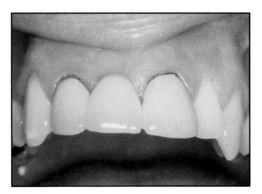

Fig. 1 Thin gingivae with resultant recession associated with a maxillary anterior bridge

Restoration of worn teeth can be made easier by surgical crown lengthening. It improves appearance and facilitates tooth preparation. Anatomical features can limit the height that can be gained.

[1]*Consultant in Restorative Dentistry, Eastman Dental Hospital, University College London Hospitals Trust and Honorary Senior Lecturer, Department of Continuing Education, Eastman Dental Institute for Oral Health Care Sciences, University of London, 256 Gray's Inn Road, London WC1X 8LD and specialist private practice, 90 Harley Street, London W1*

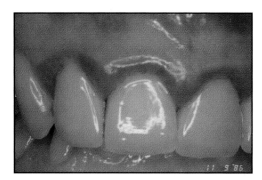

Fig. 2 Maxillary anterior crowns. Thick gingival tissue showing chronic inflammation

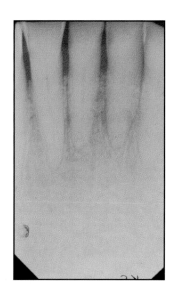

Fig. 3 Radiograph showing cylindrical teeth

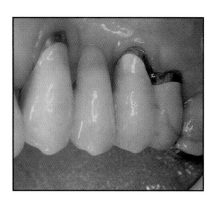

Fig. 4 Metal collars on porcelain fused to metal crowns

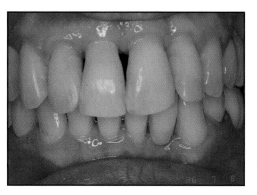

Fig. 5 Anterior view following crown lengthening surgery showing 'black triangles' between the teeth

lengthening. These factors include:

- The shape of single-rooted teeth
- The size of embrasure space and lip height
- Molar root morphology
- The width of interdental bone
- Muscle insertions
- Soft tissue aesthetics.

Shape of single-rooted teeth

In order to fabricate metal-ceramic crowns it is generally necessary to remove a minimum of 1.3 mm of tooth to accommodate the restorative material. In thin teeth, because of the narrowness of the dentine at the level of the amelo-cemental junction it may not be possible to reduce the tooth by such an amount without either exposing the pulp or leaving the technician insufficient width to accommodate the materials used for a metal-ceramic crown. This results in over-contouring compromising plaque control.

Where single-rooted teeth tend to be cylindrical (fig. 3), if there is sufficient room at the level of the amelo-cemental junction to make the preparation, then extending the length of the clinical crown in an apical direction will still allow a reasonable crown preparation to be made. If there is insufficient room at the amelo-cemental junction, or if the tooth tapers significantly from that point, then metal-ceramic crowns can only be used without overcontouring if they have metal cervical collars. These require bevelled margins which need less tooth reduction in the marginal areas (fig. 4). The use of a metal collar has aesthetic implications if the patient has a high lip-line.

Size of embrasure space and lip height

Where the tooth root tapers from the amelo-cemental junction to the apex, after crown lengthening the post-surgical aesthetics may be poor because of the appearance of the very wide embrasure spaces that leave black triangles between the teeth (fig. 5). This will be especially noticeable where the patient has a high lip-line. This effect can be partially reduced by either modifying the surgical technique in order to preserve the papilla or by over-building the neck of the crowns to reduce the size of the interdental area. The latter is difficult to do without compromising plaque removal.

Molar root morphology

Single-rooted conical posterior teeth can be treated like anterior teeth provided the root does not have marked developmental grooves. Removing bone from the coronal end of a groove may leave gutters along which plaque can track in an apical direction. If this is anticipated odontoplasty may be required to eliminate them.

Deliberate bone removal around multi-rooted teeth can result in exposure of the furcation entrance leading to problems in plaque control which may encourage future loss of bone. Where a tooth has a short root 'trunk', crown lengthening all around the tooth will not be feasible. This is a diagnosis made from a radiograph (fig. 6). In this situation it may be possible to remove bone from the mesial and distal regions of a lower molar without compromising bone in the furcation area. This is less than ideal but may still be useful. If the radiograph (fig. 7) shows the tooth has a long root 'trunk', provided the need to maintain 3 mm. width between the most apical extension of the crown and the crest of the alveolar bone is recognised, bone may be removed around the circumference of the tooth.

A similar problem may exist in premolar teeth, especially in the maxillary arch. About 40 per cent of first maxillary premolar teeth have two roots, one buccal and one palatal. The result of this is a mesio-distal bi-furcation. Even if there are not two distinct roots, there may be a very distinct groove, usually on the mesial aspect. When removing bone, ideally it should be removed interdentally to give not only increased clinical crown height on the proximal surfaces but also to allow sufficient room for the re-positioned interdental soft tissue. In the multi-rooted bicuspid, it may not be possible to satisfy these aims.

Width of interdental bone

When extending the height of the clinical crown it is not sufficient to remove bone only on the buccal or labial surface. It must also be removed interproximally as well as lingually or palatally. Failure to remove interdental bone may compromise the increase in crown height and consequently retention and resistance form of the restoration as well as leaving insufficient room to accommodate the interdental soft tissue.

If a pre-operative radiograph shows very narrow interdental bone as a consequence of there being little space between adjacent teeth (fig. 8) it may be impossible to use instruments, either hand or rotary, to remove the interdental bone without damaging the adjacent tooth surfaces. In this situation consideration should be given to whether removal of the tooth and replacement with a pontic might be preferable.

Muscle insertions

The depth of the vestibular fornix is determined by the underlying muscles. For example, in the mandibular anterior region, mentalis muscle is inserted at the maximum concavity of the labial surface of the mandible. When apically re-positioning a muco-gingival flap after bone removal to partially expose the root of the tooth, the space available to accommodate the flap is determined by the muscle insertion. A shallow vestibule due to the attachment of buccinator and mentalis muscles limits the space available to accommodate the re-positioned

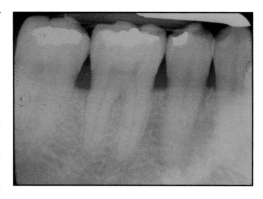

Fig. 6 Radiograph of a mandibular first molar showing a 'short trunk'

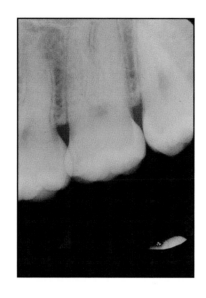

Fig. 7 Radiograph of a maxillary first molar showing a 'long trunk'

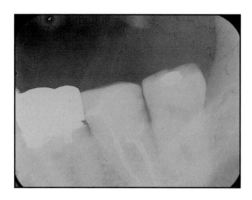

Fig. 8 Radiograph showing thin interdental bone between three mandibular molars

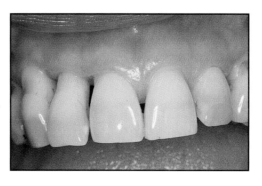

Fig. 9 View of maxillary anterior teeth showing unacceptable aesthetics

muco-gingival flap which will in turn limit the amount of coronal extension possible. This is particularly a problem in those patients with an Class II occlusion. The nearer the gonial angle is to 90° the shallower will be the depth of the mandibular fornix in the anterior region.

Soft tissue — aesthetic considerations

Substantial re-contouring around a single tooth is rarely aesthetically successful in areas which show on smiling. Following healing, the contrast in soft tissue shape between the treated tooth and the untreated adjacent teeth may be noticeable, especially in the mid-line. A minimum of two central incisor teeth and often all six anterior teeth may need to be crown lengthened so as to produce acceptable aesthetics (fig. 9). If only one tooth requires crown lengthening, in order to gain even gingival heights, consideration should be given to forced eruption by means of orthodontics which is then followed by surgery. The latter is important to re-establish normal gingival contour as the periodontal attachment is erupted along with the tooth.

Following surgery, the gingival margin will not heal to its final position for 20 weeks. Wise showed that following crown lengthening procedures there was initially coronal movement of the marginal tissue following which there was apical shrinkage which continued until 20 weeks after surgery.[3] Therefore, if restorations are to be placed with their margins just sub-gingival, it is prudent to wait until 6 months after surgery to be certain that no further change in the position of the gingival margin takes place.

Having analysed all the anatomical factors and decided on the amount of crown lengthening that is possible, if the clinician undertaking the restorative stage of treatment is not the same person who will undertake the surgery, it is essential that this information is communicated by trimming a set of stone casts to show the surgeon the final tissue contour required.

Finally, crown lengthening procedures, where the tissue is healthy, hurt! It is an essential part of treatment planning that the patient should be advised of this prior to surgery, so pain control measures can be undertaken. They should be advised pain does not indicate poor healing. Transient tooth mobility may occur and the use of a periodontal dressing on the labial and buccal surfaces is normal. This may mean scheduling appointments to fit in with social engagements.

Surgical crown lengthening procedures can form an essential adjunct to the restorative management of teeth affected by tooth surface loss. There are occasions when the restorative procedures cannot be completed without them. A previous paper in this series showed how orthodontic treatment could be of assistance in creating interocclusal space prior to restorative procedures in people with worn teeth. Periodontal surgery is another adjunctive procedure that must be considered at an early stage in planning restorative care. It is one of the frequently indicated strategies for assisting in creating adequate mechanical, occlusal and aesthetics outcomes in restorative treatment. The final article in this series will deal with reconstruction of the dentition damaged by tooth surface loss such that conservative methods are not appropriate.

1 Gargiulo A, Wentz F M, Orban B. Dimensions and relations of the dentogingival junction in humans. *J Periodontol* 1961; **32**: 261-267.
2 Cohen D W. Current approaches to periodontology. *J Periodontol* 1964; **35**: 5-18.
3 Wise M D. Stability of gingival crest after surgery and before anterior crown placement. *J Prosthet Dent* 1985; **53**: 20-23.

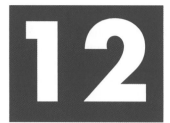

12 Conventional crown and bridgework

D. J. Setchell[1]

In considering the contribution of 'conventional' cemented fixed prosthodontic restorations to the management of extensively worn dentitions, immediately we are confronted with a paradox. It would be challenging to explain to someone who is not a dentist how a treatment modality traditionally dependent on the removal of substantial amounts of coronal tooth tissue could possibly be appropriate for a patient whose main presenting difficulty is excessive loss of just that precious commodity.

Preceding articles in the series have emphasised the need for prevention and the strategies that may used. Part 5 described the more attractive options for replacing what has been lost using 'adhesive' restorations that are inherently more conservative. These are undoubtedly preferable where sufficient enamel and dentine remains for them to perform well. They have transformed the management of many patients who would previously have required traditional indirect restorations. Nevertheless, there remain some for whom appearance and function can be provided most efficiently with cemented restorations. Reconstructions of this type have a proven record of long service. They require a different set of strategies from those employed where teeth are relatively unworn. It is those strategies, rather than the technical details of construction, which are discussed in this article.

The nature of the problem
The first paper in the series discussed the nature of tooth wear. However, we need to revise those aspects which directly affect treatment planning for cemented restorations and to highlight the problems that will result if techniques that were learned for the restora-

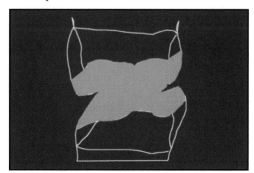

Fig. 1 Volume and distribution of tissue lost during wear

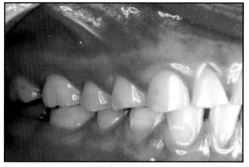

Fig. 2 Compensation accompanying tooth surface loss

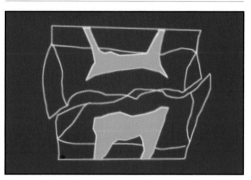

Fig. 3 Wear resulting in pulps almost in occlusion

tion of 'normal' teeth are applied in a case of extensive tooth wear.

Where teeth are unworn, the crown heights are favourable and the pulps separated by a volume of enamel and dentine that could easily accommodate tooth reduction for crowns without undue risk. The axial walls of the preparation could offer good retention and resistance form while sufficient dentine would remain to give the preparation mechanical strength. Figure 1 is an outline showing the extent of tooth loss that might be found in a worn dentition. If only the lost tissue left a space it would be a relatively easy task to replace the missing tooth tissue with an onlay of some kind to restore function and appearance. Unfortunately, it is unusual to find such a case.

The effects of tooth wear
In a patient of the kind shown in figure 2, all the results of the compensatory effects that accompany progressive wear are seen. Although the pulps are likely to have deposited a great deal of secondary dentine and may well be 'stressed' as a result of the insults they have had to tolerate, the situation is likely to be that

[1] Senior Lecturer and Head of Department of Conservative Dentistry, Eastman Dental Institute for Oral Health Care Sciences. University of London and Honorary Consultant in Restorative Dentistry, Eastman Dental Hospital, University College London Hospital Trust

The restorations of worn teeth with crowns requires a number of strategies to create space for retentive, resistant and durable castings

shown in figure 3. There is no room to work between the pulp chambers any more. Compensation has advanced the teeth into the 'occlusal interface' to maintain functional contact as wear occurs. The entire dentition has remodelled to eliminate the space we require for restoration. Only a brave man would consider attempting to prepare these teeth according to standard fixed prosthodontic methods. To do so would result in short, wide preparations lacking retention and resistance, a high risk of further pulpal injury, and restorations of bizarre occlusal form and appearance. They would tend to be very thin, and both dentist and technician would struggle: unfortunately, they often do.

Where did the space go ?

There are several physiological responses which have happened progressively over a long period and may be hard to perceive. Continuing 'tooth eruption' is certainly one, but unlike the eruption that takes place in a developing dentition it tends not to propel the teeth 'out' of the alveolar process. Unless periodontal disease is present, the attachment apparatus remodels with slow tooth movement, leaving the mucogingival line in its original position and producing a widened zone of attached gingiva. The clinical crowns are shortened: the roots of teeth tend to taper, so a narrower part comes to occupy the marginal zone and the tissues overlying the roots may be thick. These changes may give the appearance of robust periodontal support and perhaps explain the old adage that patients with 'hog's gums' have a tendency to tooth wear. The converse is probably nearer the truth.

Meanwhile there is cemental apposition on the root surfaces, remodelling of the alveoli, some shallowing of the socket depths, mesial drift and possibly other fine positional changes all 'designed' to preserve functional capacity as the teeth wear. There is potential for an altered jaw relationship which may bring wider parts of the mandibular arch to oppose narrower parts of the maxillary arch and so distort bucco-lingual and antero-posterior relations.

Occlusal changes

Many clinicians assume that there is a reduction in occlusal vertical dimension (OVD) and an increase in 'freeway space'. In fact the lower third face height may be affected less than they believe. This is a discussion that is academically interesting but only marginally relevant to treatment.

So far as the individual teeth are concerned, wear may result in a wide range of changes depending on the aetiology and the original occlusal relationship. Moreover, the wear may be generalised , tending to affect all of the teeth, or it may be localised so that part of the dentition compensates but other parts do not. There may thus be a lot of change in the overall occlusal scheme, or local changes superimposed on what was originally present.

Typically the cuspal anatomy of posterior teeth is lost and the supporting cusps wear more extensively than the non-supporting ones (fig. 4). The characteristic narrowing of the intact occlusal table maintained by the supporting cusp shape is lost. Combined with the other compensatory changes described, this may result in broad, flat teeth having close to an 'end-to-end' relationship (fig. 5). The non-supporting cusps can no longer keep the soft tissues away from the contacts between supporting cusps, so that the patient may well begin to bite his cheek or tongue. The axial surfaces may also be damaged. Clearly, appropriate

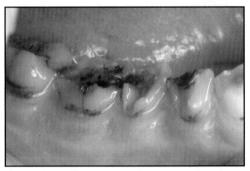

Fig. 4 Wear affects supporting cusps more than non-supporting

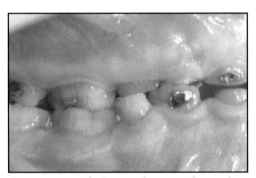

Fig. 5 Wear producing an almost 'end-to-end' relationship of the teeth

occlusal anatomy cannot be restored unless the teeth can be 'disengaged' enough to put back a sensible occlusal scheme.

Anteriorly, much will depend on the relationship before wear took place. There is a tendency for anterior guidance relationships to be lost so that increasing amounts of posterior tooth contact occur in excursive movements. This fuels the attritional component of the wear process, leading to fractures of weakened teeth or restorations.

The most striking effects occur when wear exposes extensive areas of dentine on maxillary palatal surfaces to the moving edges of the enamel 'plates' of lower teeth, developing the adverse type of relationship from a restorative point of view depicted in figure 6.

There are as many individual variations in pattern as there are patients. Figure 7 shows a man

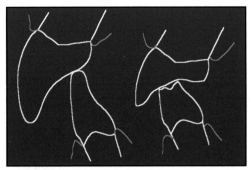

Fig. 6 Unworn and severely worn anterior teeth

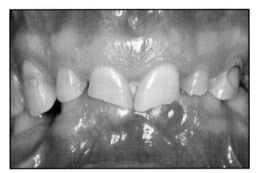

Fig. 7 Severely worn anterior teeth

with virtually no wear of posterior teeth, but in whom extensive wear and compensation have affected the anterior segments. What is left of the lower incisors occludes with the secondary dentine deposited within the original root canals.

In the Class II division 1 jaw relation prevalent in UK, there can be extensive loss of palatal tissue from the maxillary incisors before appearance is much affected and the patient seeks help. If the mandibular incisors are relatively intact, this will simplify treatment. Where they are not, a particularly difficult challenge will be faced trying to restore the functional incisal edges of these small teeth with an acceptable material. The fact that maxillary incisors are so often restored with ceramic materials may lead to localised wear of their antagonists, a feature that only becomes cause for complaint when the restorations require replacement or the lower teeth are almost worn away.

At the diagnostic stage of management the clinician may well wonder what malign influence has conspired to produce a worn occlusion that seems specifically *designed* to make his life difficult. There is a rational explanation based on the plethora of factors that influence local wear rates: action of erosive agents and buffering effects, the cross-sectional size of the teeth, occlusal contact relations, the nature of the surfaces involved, parafunctional activities, habits and almost certainly more that are not understood.

Decisions

The hardest decision for the dental practitioner to make ought to be straightforward, but clearly is not. A tooth wear case in which conventional crowns and bridges are contemplated is likely to be one in which opportunities for early intervention have passed. The wear, and thus the compensation for it, are almost certainly advanced. The decision is to decide that a satisfactory result cannot be achieved without using one or more of the strategies that are now described.

The teeth and supporting structures must be evaluated carefully as in any other fixed prosthodontic case, but the primary need is to *determine how we are to achieve space for restorative material* with only a minimum of further tooth reduction. Attention must be focussed on overcoming, or better still reversing, the effects of the compensation that has occurred: it has taken years to happen and may take a relatively long time to manage. Patients understand this if it is thoughtfully explained; sometimes it appears that we do not .

Strategies

The practising dentist naturally tends to cling to the jaw relationship and tooth positions that are present on initial examination. The common term for this is a *conformative* approach to restoration. There is nothing wrong with this if we can provide aesthetic, functional restorations for a few teeth rapidly without compromising retention and resistance form of the preparations or undertaking destructive preparation. The greater the wear, the more difficult this becomes.

So how could more space be obtained to correct tooth relationships for a fixed solution?

Occlusal equilibration

It is always possible that the patient has acquired a slide between the retruded contact position (RCP) and the intercuspal position (ICP) that requires them to close with the anterior teeth in an adverse relation. The posterior teeth may also be difficult to restore in the ICP, which is apt to change as tooth preparations are performed. The practitioner with awareness of functional occlusion may decide to obtain relaxation of the masticatory musculature by a period of occlusal splint therapy and investigate the feasibility of adjusting some of the natural teeth to secure a more favourable working jaw relation. A clinical example of this was provided in Part 10 of the series.

Adjustment alone rarely provides a solution in cases of advanced wear, since it is difficult to establish a definite intercuspal position in a more distal relationship by equilibration. It is also hard to justify to a patient with wear that one is intending to grind teeth that may already be sensitive. In more than 20 years of specialist practice, the author can remember only a handful of wear cases in which adjustment *alone* was effective before localised restoration. It is more often used as a pre-restorative measure before extensive restoration.

A working knowledge of occlusal methods more frequently suggests a combination of stabilisation of the occlusion in RAP with the measure that for many years has been *force majeure* in management of the of generalised tooth wear. That is of course increasing the occlusal vertical dimension (OVD), a method that generates considerable controversy.

Increasing the occlusal vertical dimension — reorganisation

At a time before the ease of obtaining relative axial movement of groups of teeth was appreciated, disengagement of a 'close' occlusal relationship to permit restoration was seen to require an overall approach to reconstruction. Many, or even all, of the teeth in at least one arch were restored, usually to provide a final occlusion in which ICP was re-established coincident with RAP. The term *'reorganisation'* came to be applied to this strategy, though an increase in contact OVD in retruded axis position is not necessarily implied. Raising the OVD may provide enough interocclusal space to largely eliminate occlusal reduction when preparing the teeth thus preserving axial wall height that is often at a premium. Unfortunately, it separates the anterior teeth by a factor of 3× the posterior separation and this can be embarrassing if the anterior teeth already looked long enough and did not have much vertical overlap.

How well is it tolerated ?

Here a digression is required to note that many authorities, often with a removable prosthodontic background, have held serious reservations about the safety of any change in the contact OVD of a natural dentition. The doubt arises from concern that the patient may not be able to 'tolerate' the increase. We read often of the need to test any proposed increase with preliminary diagnostic appliances. More often than not, these appliances, rather than the increased OVD, are difficult to tolerate. Given that a stable intercuspal position can be provided in the new relationship, an acceptable anterior guidance is achieved and posterior cuspal interference is eliminated, the author has never encountered a case in which a judicious increase in OVD was not instantly accepted. Moreover, there is a conceptual difference between such an increase in a tooth or implant-supported occlusion and the denture equivalent. If we increase the contact OVD of a tooth-supported dentition it is likely that the lower third face height will be increased at the time the restorations are inserted. If, several years later, the teeth occlude in an unchanged way but alveolar remodelling has returned the lower third face height to its original dimension, have we 'increased the OVD' or not ? The author does not mind, as long as we have gained space to restore the teeth conservatively. One cannot apply the same arguments to complete dentures where care of the denture-bearing ridges is paramount.

It is suggested that terms such as 'restoring the OVD' be deleted from the vocabulary as confusing. We increase it, perhaps temporarily.

Much the same arguments apply to 'freeway space'. It may well be a significant diagnostic factor in denture construction, but what evidence there is suggests that the dentate individual assumes a new rest position in response to the ICP that is provided.

There are enough real problems in fixed prosthodontics for us to avoid inventing virtual ones. Any change in OVD of a natural dentition large enough to cause a problem with freeway space would long before have resulted in a ridiculous anterior tooth relationship.

Case study — increasing the OVD

Figure 8 shows a female patient treated at the Eastman from the late 1970s and is used to show how increasing the OVD was performed at a time when caution was the watchword. The posterior teeth had advanced wear, but the mandibular anteriors were less severely affected. Figure 9 shows the left side in ICP and the limited crown height available for restorations. The maxillary teeth had adequate buccal height but had lost their palatal (supporting) cusps. Figure 10 shows that a modest increase in OVD transformed the feasibility of restoration.

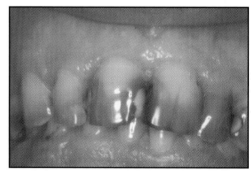

Fig. 8 Dentition which showed severe wear

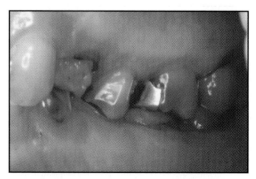

Fig. 9 Wear limiting height available for restorations

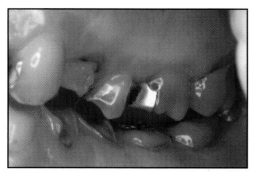

Fig. 10 Increasing OVD makes restoration feasible

A maxillary full arch splint was constructed and adjusted. After a comfortable period of wear, the anterior part of the splint was cut away and the anterior teeth to be crowned had final restorations made and inserted with temporary cement. Care was taken to develop an anterior guidance relationship that would permit disclusion of the posterior crowns later.

The posterior teeth were then prepared conserving a maximum of axial wall height, and opposing posterior sextants were restored with the results seen in figures 11 and 12, which show the canine protection selected. A graduate student thus completed the case in three relatively easy stages. It served the patient uneventfully for the rest of her life.

A commendable result, but one wonders how many such extensive reconstructions have been performed in order to provide space where there is a more localised problem? Fine treatment where it is indicated, but not otherwise. There are limits to the number of treatments of

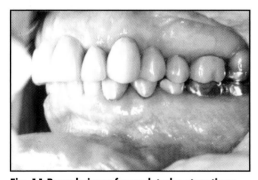

Fig. 11 Buccal view of completed restorations

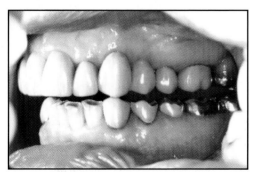

Fig. 12 The canine-protected occlusion

this kind that can be provided to a high standard. Compromise treatments using removable onlays are certainly possible, but are not as effective. These days we might have used resin-retained restorations with even less tooth reduction, but the strategy would be similar.

We therefore ask, 'What has changed?' where only a few teeth require restoration but compensation has made space a problem. There is an elegant answer, if only we have the resolve to use it:

Relative axial movement to create space
If compensatory changes have eliminated space for restorations, it should be possible to reverse the changes and re-gain the space. The dental profession owes a debt of gratitude to Dahl *et al.*[1] for showing us how effectively this can be done, but their wisdom has tended to fall on deaf ears. In the 20 years since the exposition of this simple strategy, every subsequent emulation of the original description has reiterated 'the need for more clinical trials before it can be widely adopted'. However, a recent clinical audit of 50 sequential cases at the Eastman Dental Hospital confirms yet again that it is indeed a predictable strategy. Moreover it is one that fits more easily into general dental practice than full mouth reconstruction. So what is it ?

Case study: anterior space creation
Figures 13 to 16 document an early case treated at the Eastman. A male patient in his seventies presented with a functional posterior reconstruction provided many years before by his general dental practitioner. The mandibular anterior teeth were only slightly worn, but their antagonists had extensive palatal wear through which the pulps showed pink. These teeth were hypersensitive and were enough of a problem to warrant treatment. Endodontic treatment would have eliminated the sensitivity but have done nothing to control future wear. Figure 14 shows a temporary casting cemented to the worn teeth to provide occlusal stops for the anterior teeth. A luting glass ionomer cement was used. The posteriors were separated by slightly more than the thickness required for ultimate anterior restoration. After several months of comfortable function on the anteriors only, the device was removed with the result shown on mounted casts in figure 15. There was enough space for partial coverage gold alloy restorations to be provided (fig. 16). It would have been gratuitous to provide full coverage and remove what useful structure had survived.

In the intervening 18 years this strategy has become an everyday aid. Similar results are obtainable with composite resin additions. Young patients respond quickly since the teeth that are separated erupt while those in contact are intruded. Those of us who are older may take many months to achieve useful space because intrusion is the main response.

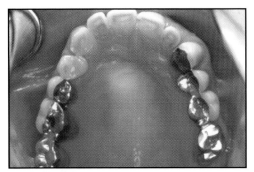

Fig. 13 Stable posterior dentition, severely worn anteriors

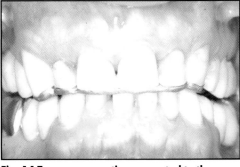

Fig. 14 Temporary casting cemented to the anterior teeth

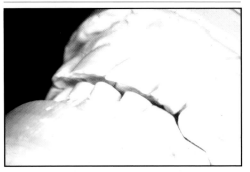

Fig. 15 Casts showing space created

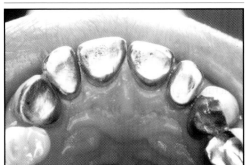

Fig. 16 Teeth restored with partial coverage gold restorations

The method also works well for posterior teeth. Figures 17 to 20 show a female patient with erosion and missing maxillary molars. The lower first molar had erupted into contact with the opposing alveolus. Temporary nickel-chrome bridges placed these teeth in contact at an increased vertical dimension. As intrusion occurred, composite resin was added to maintain supraocclusion until the lower occlusal plane was corrected (fig. 19). The final bridge is shown in figure 20, intrusion of the upper abutments eliminating the need for occlusal reduction. Follow-up for ten years has confirmed no adverse consequences for any of the teeth treated.

The results of this strategy are such that it is no longer justifiable to run the risk of preparing worn teeth to obtain interocclusal space when it is readily available by other means. Moreover, there is no need to sacrifice crown height that is required for retention and resistance. Nor is it a common procedure any more to electively devitalise teeth so that post/core restorations

can be placed to extend short clinical crowns. Once we have explored why this is true, we have all of the strategic tools that will enable almost all wear cases to be satisfactorily restored.

Surgical crown lengthening

Since the periodontal tissues in health accompany the teeth as they migrate occlusally during compensatory movements, it is sometimes necessary to resect alveolar bone and establish sufficient clinical crown height for restoration. This procedure is no help at all with the occlusal complications of tooth wear, but it has three important contributions:

Gingival contour: Periodontal surgery may place the gingival level of teeth into harmony with those that have worn less, avoiding a 'gummy' result with short, square restorations.

Axial wall height: Dentine that was formerly subgingival or within alveolar bone may be converted into 'clinical crown' and is rendered accessible for preparation. The final restoration can

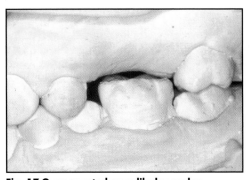

Fig. 17 Over-erupted mandibular molar

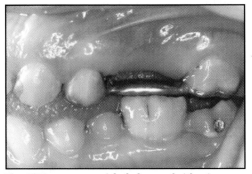

Fig. 18 Temporary nickel-chrome bridge in maxillary arch

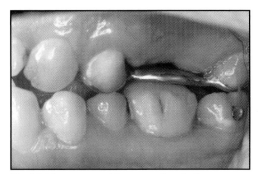

Fig. 19 The corrected lower occlusal plane

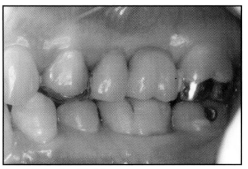

Fig. 20 The final bridge

thus have enhanced retention and resistance.

Structural strength: What remains of the tooth supragingivally may be extensively weakened, particularly where previous restorations were present. The operator must consider how much structural dentine will remain in the preparations after axial reduction and be aware that it may fracture after a crown has been cemented. Crown lengthening will uncover 'new' sound dentine to form a structural foundation.

Case study: surgical crown lengthening and reorganisation

Figure 21 shows a male patient with *dentinogenesis imperfecta* which had resulted in very advanced tooth wear early in adult life. This man does not have a Class III malocclusion, despite appearances. He shows all of the effects previously described. His buccal occlusion was illustrated in figure 5. Crown lengthening was required in all areas of the mouth and figure 22 shows the anterior view after surgery. The surgery has achieved all three effects just described, but an increase in OVD and reorganisation of the occlusal scheme so that RCP and ICP were made coincident were also necessary to achieve the results depicted in figure 23.

The considerations for surgical crown lengthening were discussed in Part 11 of the series.

This paper has provided an overview of the treatment strategies that may be enlisted to convert the apparently untreatable case of advanced tooth wear into one where conventional crown and bridge procedures can prove successful. Treatment is based on an accurate diagnosis of the problems that the wear has produced. In circumstances where significant compensation for the tooth surface loss has taken place, the most appropriate strategy is likely to include relative axial tooth movement to reverse the compensatory changes.

This series has provided a detailed account of many aspects of tooth surface loss. It is appropriate that it ends with the description of the role of conventional crown and bridge highlighting the complexities of such work. This reinforces the need for alertness, early diagnosis and the establishment of effective preventive

regimes in patients showing early signs of tooth surface loss: there do remain however considerable difficulties in monitoring their effectiveness. Consequently physical methods for protecting the teeth form part of such programmes. Adhesive restorations sometimes placed early in the process of erosive wear should be considered part of this strategy.

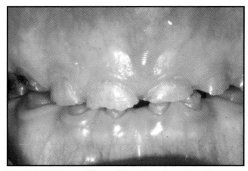

Fig. 21 Patient affected by *dentinogenesis imperfecta*

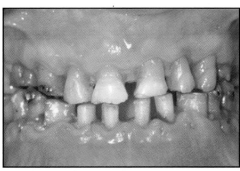

Fig. 22 Following surgical crown lengthening

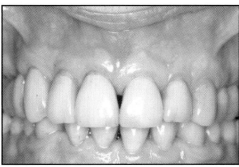

Fig. 23 The final restorative result

1. Dahl B L, Krogstad O K, Karlsen K. An alternative treatment in cases with advanced localized attrition. *J Oral Rehab* 1975; 2: 209-214.

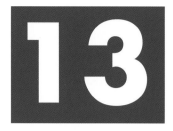

Tooth surface loss: future considerations

R. Ibbetson, and A. Eder

The introduction outlined the widespread nature of the problem of tooth surface loss. It highlighted the difficulties of diagnosis, controlling the progression of wear and the difficulties that arise when restoration of the teeth becomes necessary. The series set out to address some of the issues of aetiology, diagnosis and treatment. However, there are aspects of the management of patients that remain problematical.

Diagnosis and monitoring wear
Successful management will continue to require correct identification of the primary aetiology. Without this, care is likely to be inappropriate and wear progressive. The interaction and inter-relation between erosion, abrasion and attrition complicates diagnosis. Unfortunately identification of the primary aetiology is sometimes difficult requiring care in the history-taking and a careful analysis of the appearance of the teeth. Even when the nature of the tooth surface loss is understood, in cases of acid erosion the precise aetiological factors can be difficult to determine: this in turn can make preventive management difficult. The type of tooth wear does not necessarily present a consistent clinical picture. A dentition affected primarily by acid erosion is likely also to show evidence of wear brought about by tooth-to-tooth contact: while bruxist activity may produce characteristic features to which can be added elements of tooth surface loss caused by an erosive process.

In patients affected by wear, elimination of the aetiologic cause may not prevent continued wear as when enamel has been lost, the less hard dentine may continue to wear through a process of simple abrasion of the occlusal surfaces during function. This requires that the effectiveness of preventive strategies is reviewed at regular intervals. Unfortunately monitoring whether wear is progressive can be exceptionally difficult. The techniques available are at best primitive and only likely to yield information when significant further loss of tooth tissue has taken place. The indices that are currently available have not gained acceptance as being useful in their clinical application.

The essential problem is that as the dentition wears, there is little that remains stable which can act as a reference against which assessment of progression can be made. Continued eruption of the teeth takes place in order to maintain occlusal contact between antagonists whilst the position of the gingival margin cannot be considered fixed. As continued eruption takes place, the alveolar housing and the gingivae move with the tooth but changes in gingival health and in the morphology of the alveolar bone around the teeth may permit an element of apical migration of the junctional epithelium or a change in form of the marginal gingival tissues. Simple viewing of serial study casts is therefore suspect whilst changes in the form of the teeth or the soft tissues make reproducible location of matrices made from earlier casts or directly intra-orally suspect. The only useful fixed points are Class V restorations and the decreased incidence of dental caries makes it increasingly less likely that these may be available as reference points. It is said that in cases of acid erosion, continued sensitivity may be an indication that wear is continuing but such statements are at best based on clinical experience and at worst are anecdotal.

In conclusion, re-assessment requires that further history taking is combined with clinical observation, review of study casts and the use of indices. However, the absence of detectable ongoing wear does not necessarily mean that it has ceased. Wear of 200 micrometres a year is likely to have clinical significance but is unlikely to be detectable unless the patient is reviewed over extended periods against base-line records. It is therefore important, as described in Part 6, that the patient is given their base-line casts to counter the effects of patient and dentist migration.

Much of the series focused on acid dissolution of teeth as it has emerged as one of the modern dental diseases. However, in many ways it is easier to manage than tooth surface loss resultant from bruxist activity. The latter has been identified for many years as a cause not only of tooth wear but also as producing increased loads on teeth and restorations with a capability of damaging both. The aetiology of

The series has discussed the aetiology and management of tooth surface loss. However, there remain aspects that require research and greater understanding if the care of patients is to be improved.

parafunctional activity has never been identified to the point where a primary preventive strategy has been established which can eliminate the problem. Current approaches aim to prevent the ill-effects of prolonged and sustained loading of teeth or restorations. The provision of an occlusal splint as described in Part 3 remains the only absolutely reliable way of controlling the effects. The role of occlusal adjustment once favoured in minimising or eliminating bruxist activity has been diminished by a lack of supporting scientific evidence to the point where it has little or no part to play in a preventive strategy. Dentists demand much of their patients in asking them to cooperate in a strategy that requires them to wear an appliance indefinitely. There is perhaps more chance of their doing so if the patient considers the wear to be a problem or if they have invested significant time and money in having previously worn teeth restored. Patients with teeth worn due to parafunctional activity must be counselled as to the long-term benefits of an occlusal splint and the potential consequences of not wearing one. It requires sustained motivation by both the patient and the members of the clinical dental team.

The series has also stressed the need to use restorative materials that will not promote tooth wear. The development of newer ceramics and composite resins has already started to reduce the severity of this problem. Nevertheless selection of materials still requires care. The use of ceramic materials on the functional surfaces of teeth affected by erosion should be avoided whilst ceramic on anterior guidance surfaces in bruxists is also likely to promote further wear.

It is perhaps cervical abrasion that is the least worrying of all the types of tooth surface loss. There is a frequently perceived association between inappropriate oral hygiene practices and its presence. However, in clinical practice this does not always seem to be the case. Such lesions might be due to abfraction where occlusal forces are resolved such that stress is concentrated in the buccal cervical area of the teeth. Such a concept has support in the dental literature. However, in these times of an evidence-based approach to treatment, cause and effect has not been demonstrated and occlusal adjustment as a method for preventing cervical abrasion cavities cannot be justified. Management of these lesions must remain with ensuring that tooth cleaning is appropriate and making conservative adhesive restorations if necessary, as described in Part 5 of this series. These can prevent loss of tooth structure cervically that might compromise the structural integrity of the crown of the tooth.

A further theme that runs through this text is consideration of the preventive restoration of teeth. It has been said that no restorations should be made until the cause of the wear has been identified and the aetiological factors controlled. This principle is correct. However sometimes the cause of tooth surface loss, particularly that caused by acid erosion, can resist diagnosis. Wear of the palatal surfaces of the maxillary anterior teeth often leads to thinning of the incisal edges which then begin to chip. When this is seen, early restoration using conservative methods such as adhesive resins or adhesive indirect restorations should be considered as continued wear may produce a significant aesthetic deficit which in turn may require more extensive restoration. Such restorations were described in detail in Parts 5 and 8. These conservative restorations particularly those made of composite resin can be considered similar in concept to the preventive resin restoration, now an accepted part of the management of carious lesions in posterior teeth.

Methods of restoration

Traditional crown and bridgework techniques are destructive of remaining tooth structure. Their use requires an assessment of both the short-term and long-term sequelae and is a balance between gain and loss. The worn tooth presents a number of problems which frequently mean that traditional crowns may not be appropriate. Successful crowns require that sufficient space is generated occlusally and axially to create an adequate functional surface for occlusal stability with enough thickness to contribute to rigidity and resist wear leading to perforation. Sufficient axial wall height is necessary to create good retention and resistance form which will protect the cement lute from degradation and breakdown. The requirements can be difficult to satisfy and strategies for enhancing the availability of sufficient inter-occlusal clearance and adequate axial wall height were described in Parts 9 and 12.

Developments in adhesive restorations used both directly and indirectly will continue. The series has already described their preferable use in the worn dentition affected by acid erosion. Clinicians should assess the feasibility of this approach in every instance as the advantages are clear: they simplify clinical procedures and lessen tooth morbidity. Techniques for creating space for restoring worn teeth have also changed, many authors in the series described the role of relative axial tooth movement. This method has been slow to be taken up within the setting of primary dental care, perhaps not surprisingly given its implications for the traditionally controversial areas of raising the vertical dimension of occlusion and localised occlusion on small groups of teeth. It is worth remembering that it was first recorded nearly twenty-five years ago and has been frequently described over the years. The method should be part of routine dental care as the alternatives are generally more costly, complicated and destructive.

At the same time that developments in dental materials continue, advances are needed in the diagnosis and prevention of acid erosion. Health education has been successful in changing people's diets and the attitudes of many to tobacco and alcohol. The trend towards healthier living may have inadvertently exposed people to an increased risk of suffering from tooth wear. The dental team has a major role to play in informing their patients of ways to avoid tooth surface loss.

Index

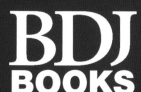

TOOTH SURFACE LOSS

The management of individuals suffering from tooth surface loss can be difficult and time consuming.

Tooth Surface Loss addresses those difficulties by providing practical, clinical techniques to help dentists identify the aetiological factors responsible for erosion, abrasion and attrition and offers assistance in planning and delivering appropriate patient care. The book covers the difficulties encountered in diagnosis and prevention of tooth surface loss, problems associated with controlling the process and strategies for providing restorative solutions.

- Eating disorders and the dentist
- Occlusion and splint therapy
- Removable prostheses
- Adhesive techniques
- Prevention and maintenance
- Dealing with failures

- Tooth wear in the child and youth
- Treatment planning
- Orthodontic options
- Surgical crown lengthening
- Conventional crown and bridgework

Tooth Surface Loss is the only book currently available covering the subject area in such a practical way. Liberally illustrated, Tooth Surface Loss, is written by clinicians who include restorative dentists and other specialists reflecting the frequent need for inter-disciplinary care for tooth surface loss patients

The emphasis throughout is on practical, clinical techniques. An essential guide for general dental practitioners, senior dental undergraduates and postgraduates.

ISBN 0 904 588 661

ISBN 0-904-588-661

9 780904 588668

BD BOOK